D0339648

Healing Sick Houses

Dowsing for Healthy Homes

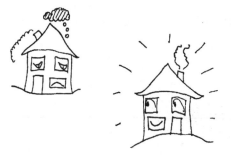

Roy and Ann Procter

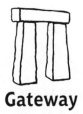

Gateway

Gateway
an imprint of
Gill & Macmillan Ltd
Hume Avenue
Park West
Dublin 12
with associated companies throughout the world
www.gillmacmillan.ie

© 2000 Roy and Ann Procter
0 7171 2992 6
Index compiled by Alick Bartholomew
Print origination by Alanna Corballis
Printed by ColourBooks Ltd, Dublin

A catalogue record is available for this book
from the British Library.

1 3 5 4 2

Dedication

from Ann to Roy
and from Roy to Ann
recognising that our forty-six-year marriage
has provided the foundation for this book.

CONTENTS

Acknowledgements

Bruce MacManaway started us off on all this, bless him. We are so glad that Patricia, his widow and Patrick, his son, have encouraged us to *stay tuned*. We acknowledge gratefully all the teachers, students, clients and associates who have provided us with more opportunities and insights over the years. In the crucial weeks before bringing this publication to fruition, we thank our good friend Alick Bartholomew, publisher extraordinary, for keeping us on track. We are most grateful to Sig Lonegren, respected long-term teacher and colleague, who made invaluable contributions when we missed seeing the wood for the trees; to our daughter Ruth, for looking at the manuscript and making suggestions in short order; and to our daughter Jane, who drew the pictures of the sad and happy houses which became our logo. The book has gained immeasurably from the personal stories in Chapter 7, and we thank those contributors most warmly.

FOREWORD

by Sig Lonegren

The uses of dowsing have exploded in the last thirty years. My mother taught me to dowse in the late fifties, but it wasn't until the early seventies that I began to work with geomancy and dowsing seriously. At that time, ninety-nine out of a hundred people had probably never heard of the word *dowsing*, and if they had, they would have associated it with using a forked stick to find the spot to dig or drill for good drinking water.

Since then, awareness of the various possible ways to use dowsing has expanded dramatically. The word *dowsing* now conjures up images of oil and treasure, through health, to testing the ripeness of fruit in shops, and *yes* and *no* questions about almost anything, to its use in geomancy in sacred and secular spaces.

It was this last term, *geomancy*, that grabbed me in the early seventies. Bruce MacManaway was the man who, as far as I can tell, was a major focal point of what I would call the modern resurgence of interest in this arcane art of geomancy. Bruce became aware of his healing capabilities at Dunkirk in World War II. His wounded men were in need of medical attention. His unit had run out of medical supplies, so he used what he had: his hands. They worked. Bruce went on to become one of the best-known British healers of the twentieth century. From his Westbank Healing Centre in Strathmiglo, Fife, Scotland, Bruce began to teach others what he had learned including the fixing and healing of houses as well as individuals.

When I studied for my Masters degree in Sacred Space in the late seventies, one of my teachers was Terry Ross, who was to become President of the American Society of Dowsers. He studied with Bruce MacManaway. Roy and Ann Procter, as you will learn in this very useful book, also studied with Bruce. Even though we started at the same root — Bruce MacManaway — we travelled different paths. My geomantic work focussed on sacred space. I worked with Stonehenge, Machu Picchu and Mesa Verde, concentrating on New England's enigmatic underground stone chambers that exhibited all of the same characteristics that I found at the more famous sites. They were, like Stonehenge, oriented toward significant horizontal astronomical events. They were, like Solomon's Temple or Chartres Cathedral, constructed using sacred geometrical principles; and these chambers, mostly in my home state of Vermont, had the same pattern of earth energies — energy leys and primary underground water — that I find at pre-Protestant Reformation sacred spaces around the world.

The Procters focussed on the more secular aspects of geomancy — homes and businesses. The two fields require different skills. If you are working on someone's home, you probably won't need to know at what azimuth the Summer Solstice Sun will rise given a three degree angle of elevation in the north-eastern horizon. On the other hand, this book has many suggestions of things to do that wouldn't occur to someone building a new sacred space. There are all kinds of energies in the home that one doesn't even think about when visiting a place like Avebury.

I have developed a hypothesis that I apply when looking at dowsing results of intangible energies — such as the *earth energies* that Roy and Ann talk about. I call it *'Sig's Hypothesis Number One'* — even if they were trained by the same teacher, the chances are very good that no two dowsers will ever find the same things when dowsing for intangible targets. This is true for me in this book. Because we were trained — in effect — by the same teacher (Bruce), we actually see the principles discussed here quite similarly. Yet there are differences. For example, I put much more emphasis on primary underground water as a potential source of geopathic stress. Ann and Roy barely mention water. And that is OK, because that's the way they see it. We do each seem to ultimately see intangible things differently.

The authors have chosen to define their targets in terms, which at first concerned me because they are so general — *energy lines, power objects* and *earth energies* are three examples. I've spent most of the last thirty years attempting to be as specific as possible — *energy leys, veins of primary water* and *domes* (in Britain, some call them *blind springs*). I did this to bring these energies as close to the physical as possible. You can almost touch them. The energy that is sometimes found running concurrently with a ley has to be straight because that is at the core of the definition of a ley — a perfectly straight alignment of holy sites. Other dowsers find these veins and domes, and tap into the veins for drinking water. I felt that the ability to see straight lines across the landscape and to drill here for good drinking water somehow made these energies easier for others to see and relate to.

But, please remember that everyone finds something different. Everyone! That's why there are so many different religions with numerous subdenominations underneath. 'I stand up at this point in the service.' 'No, we devoutly believe you must be on your knees at that point!' We each see the intangible One so differently. I have come to feel that instead of lacking specificity, the energy-descriptive words the Procters have chosen to use actually make it easier for intangible dowsers like myself to follow what they're saying! An *energy line* can be anything. Every dowser I know finds lines of energy of some description or other. The same is true of *earth energies* — especially in sacred spaces — everyone finds earth energies there. A power object, is a power object, is a power object. But while these terms do mean something to each of us, they don't, no won't, look the same to each of us. So I feel the use of general terms to describe these energies in Sad Houses is actually quite liberating, and more dowsers should be able to hear the good advice that is found herein. The experienced reader will not be saying, 'No, I don't find that', because these generalised terms are almost all-inclusive. It works!

Please do not think that if you've never held a pendulum in your hand before, reading *Healing Sick Houses* will enable you to go out and be a jobbing geomancer. Dowsing instruction is given toward the end of the book, but geomantic dowsing requires a great deal of time, sensitivity and practice. On the other hand, this book delivers a solid overview of modern secular European geomancy. There are numerous examples drawn from Roy's and Ann's long career of service to healing environments. These stories not only contribute interest, but many demonstrate yet other ways one can use dowsing to heal homes that are not conducive to the health and growth of their present inhabitants.

This is a book both for beginners and active geomancers. Beginners will get the overview, a thorough picture of what's involved in working with *Sick Houses*. Active geomancers will pick up a number of useful and practical bits of solid advice.

You're in for a good read. I sure enjoyed it!

Sig Lonegren
Glastonbury, February 2000
www.geomancy.org

INTRODUCTION

Typical of a few days in our lives

The phone rings: a lady has heard that we heal sick houses. There is 'something wrong' with her home and a friend told her we could help. We try to find out more about the 'something wrong' and explain to her what we might do to put it right. We finish by undertaking to dowse her address, and let her know if our kind of healing would be appropriate. If it would be appropriate, we'll be asking her for a sketch plan of the ground floor of her house, set in its garden or immediate surroundings.

The phone rings again: a man has been to his doctor, who has tested him on a machine for allergies etc. and says he has geopathic stress. The doctor has given him our leaflet. More listening, more explanations and our usual undertaking.

And again the phone rings (Will I ever get our lunch on the table?). This person has just been away staying with a relative, and on return noticed how depressing her house felt — it was like coming into a dark fog. Her neighbour has read an article about us in a health magazine...the mixture as before.

Our mail arrives about midday. We are at the end of a long rural round. We start by sorting it into personal, earth energy jobs, read later and junk (feeling sorry for the wasted trees). This day there are two straightforward enquiries, mercifully with s.a.e., and we put our standard package in these ready for tomorrow's post.

There is a ten-page letter from a lady with longstanding ME, (*see* Glossary), who has sketched her house on the last half page. It looks more like an elevation than a floor plan and we will have to ask her for something more accurate on which to focus.

This large envelope contains detailed architects' drawings,

complete with notes about drains, and a curt note, 'We moved in six months ago and all the family has become ill. Please heal as soon as possible.'

Now a letter from someone on whose house we worked a month ago: the children were very unsettled for a few days after the healing but are now so much better than she can remember in years. The youngest is at last sleeping through the night and the other two are eating well and attending school with enthusiasm. Phew! She has sent a donation, bless her.

There is a note from a local group secretary asking us to approve a paragraph for their programme. Oh yes! — we agreed to give them a talk on our work. This always seems easy months ahead, but nearer the time the diary becomes more crowded.

More phone calls: 'Did you do our house this morning? I suddenly felt lighter after breakfast and have spent the morning clearing out the kitchen cupboards. Amazing, and I don't feel at all tired even now!' We did. Rejoicings all round.

The phone again: a national newspaper wants to interview us for their specialist complementary health page. The last time we had this kind of publicity we received over 800 enquiries, more than half wanting healing work **now**. We hadn't caught up with the backlog, so we ask the journalist to phone again in a couple of months. There is no point giving people hope that something could be done, and then making them wait ages for it to happen.

Then a worried man is on the line: he and his wife have just been to the Bristol Cancer Help Centre (where Ann used to work). They have been told by one of the doctors that there are negative earth energies through their bedroom, as detected by his dowsing. The patient's immune system is therefore being affected and her recovery compromised. An urgent job. We suggest he sends his sketch map at once. Has he access to fax? Twenty minutes later it is coming out of our machine, ready for our next healing session.

Communication systems proliferate these days. Looking up the e-mails, we find a note from a woman who came on our dowsing course, having had her home healed. She is enquiring if the house they are doing up in Provence needs this kind of subtle attention, please?

And there's a quickie 'house sold' message, with promise of donation. The place had been on the market for two years with plenty of viewers but no offers. The day after the healing a good offer was accepted and we are delighted to know that the sale is under way.

This book explains how this work developed, and the whys and wherefores of our current practice. It is a vibrant learning process, and in no way do we want the book to crystallise the work so that it is inhibited from flowing on into a lively future.

Dr Jean Hardy, writer of books on psychology, was puzzling herself about 'What is a Person?' and 'Who am I?' when it came to her that the definition could be 'I am a temporary arrangement'. This book is just that: it describes happenings, experiences, insights and thoughts along the way in developing our abilities in the healing of people and places — but it is not the last word because we are continuing that development. If you find some of our exposition lacks clarity or precision, it may be partly because of our lack of ability to express what is going on, but it is also because these matters do not lend themselves to being clear and precise. The clear and precise bits of us are used in the dowsing and healing work we do. In teaching and describing this for others we would prefer to offer what we've found, and suggest people pick up what is helpful for them in their life and work. We hope you will enjoy our stories and ideas, and the descriptions of signposts along our path, and that you find something of use to you in your own quest.

Authors' Note

Throughout this book the word 'energy' has been used as in earth energy and healing energy etc. This is because of common usage rather than being scientifically correct. We are not referring to a physical energy such as a force, electrical energy or other such forms. The 'energy' we are concerned with might be better described as 'influence' or 'information'.

Chapter 1

WHAT IS A *SICK HOUSE*?

A sick house is one in which illness, disease or lack of ease of the people who live or work there seems to be related in some way to the place. This is an oversimplified statement, as living in a particular place does not cause all our ills. There are always a number of causative factors. However, place does seem to play a significant part in many cases.

One of the clearest indications of a sick house is the reaction of people living there. We get many letters saying that the writer feels listless and drained while in the house. The effect then disappears when they go to stay somewhere else. This is often for a holiday, and the improvement is attributed to the relaxation and lack of everyday pressures. But when returning home, the feeling of lethargy returns, even if there are no significant day-to-day pressures. Lack of sleep, and a feeling of waking up tired is often associated with a sick house. This sleeplessness is some-times more marked in younger children even if the grown-ups are not affected. We often have reports of babies not sleeping well and being found squashing themselves into a corner, or at the end of their cot; they are trying to move themselves out of the influence of unhelpful energy. When the energies have been transmuted to being beneficial, the infant then sleeps better and is no longer found squashed up as before! An infant who fails to sleep affects parents by needing attention.

Children and young teenagers are often adversely affected by the energies of place more than adults. This is particularly notice-able with girls nearing puberty. The symptoms are usually lack of energy and loss of a number of days at school through illness that is sometimes not clearly defined. They may be diagnosed as having ME. There has been considerable controversy over this disease. Some say a virus causes it, others say it is a psychological problem. It could easily be both as it seems likely that the virus, of whatever sort, has not been neutralised due to the person's immune system functioning below maximum efficiency. Despite the medical name for ME being myalgic encephalomyelitis, we call it *muddled energies*. The person's own energies are being muddled by those in their surroundings and this reflects directly into the body's workings. We find that transmuting the earth energies in and under the house is often a significant factor in improving the health of such people. When these energies are positive, they encourage lifting of the spirits, and therefore an improvement in wholeness and wellbeing. The effect can be experienced in places that are already positive, such as cathedrals and places of special beauty and significance in the landscape. You feel light: this is like *levity* as opposed to gravity.

Negative earth energies are generally experienced as some kind of draining away of life-force, mostly in insidious and unconscious ways. You may notice it in everyday life when you stay for any length of time in a place that makes you depressed and heavy. It feels as if your personal battery is being flattened with no detectable cause. ME is a typical 'flat battery' disease. You can compare it to your car battery: one day when you go to start your car there is that sickening 'clunk' and no action. Someone can help to get you going with jump leads and once your alternator has done its job you can use the lights etc....and start the car again another day. And then it happens again.... Suppose the light in the boot of the car remains on after you shut the lid: you don't know it, but the energy is being drained out of the battery all the time. Removing the cause of draining, making sure the light in the boot does go out, and giving the car a better charging mechanism, will ensure it has enough power for starting, lights etc. in the future.

In the human being, changing the discharge to a positive

charge will help the body to function more efficiently, especially in its own defence, by strengthening the immune system. Dr Rosy Daniel, recent medical director of the Bristol Cancer Help Centre, in her introductory video, postulates a scale of strength of an individual's life-force (chi, ki or prana in eastern paradigms). The lower the life-force registers on her scale, the more vulnerable the person is to all kinds of disease, from outside infections such as colds and flu, to an inability to throw out mutant cancer cells from within. A reduced life-force can demonstrate itself at mental and emotional levels too: we are asked to help people with depressions, from just feeling gloomy and lethargic, to a full clinical depression needing medication and hospitalisation. It is probably what we mean when we say someone is *dispirited*; and of course a diagnosis of serious illness, or even the realisation that one is not well over a period of time, can increase this, setting up a vicious cycle.

Another way of looking at this problem is in terms of the load on a person. All sorts of things can overload our systems: stress, overwork, bad diet and too many pollutants to name just a few. If we are also being drained at a subtle level by negative earth energies or *presences* (*see* Chapter 6) our life-force lowers to the point where we are more vulnerable, and eventually reaches a point of danger and inability to cope. We hear of many people receiving healing of all kinds, feeling better for a few days, and then going downhill again: a significant clue that they might have an earth energy problem.

Research Projects

Rather more investigative work has been done in Germany and Austria into these matters than in the UK. Baron Gustav Freiherr von Pohl and other dowsers carried out an early and thorough piece of correlation in the 1920s and 1930s. Von Pohl published the results of his work and it is now available in English (*see* Bibliography and References 3.10). An example from this book concerns the town of Stettin. In the period 1910–31 there were 5,348 deaths due to cancer:

'Dr Hager, medical officer and chairman of the Medical Scientific Association in Stettin, obtained the papers of all the deaths due to cancer in the town between 1910 and 1931. Here is a summary of his accounts:

Number of Houses	Number of Cancer Deaths	Total
1,575	1	1,575
750	2	1,500
337	3	1,011
167	4	668
51	5	255
15	6	90
6	7	42
1	8	8
1	9	9
5	10 or more	190
		Total = 5,348

Table 1.1 — Cancer Deaths in Stettin 1910–31

'Dr Hager then took the trouble to consult a dowser, privy counsellor C. William, and the two of them went to all the above houses and found that under each house was an underground current and under some, where underground streams crossed, which were very strong indeed.

'Especially interesting and informative was the result in the old people's homes, because as Dr Hager explained in his talk to the medical association, there were old people of the same vulnerability to cancer.

'The one home stands above a cross of underground currents and is completely radiated. In 21 years, 28 cancer deaths occurred.

'The second home had, during the same period, two cases. The home is radiated only by two small underground currents, and Dr Hager discovered that the deceased had their beds exactly above these lines.

'In the third home there was not one cancer case in more than 20 years. The investigation concluded that there were no underground currents.'

This sort of data certainly makes one think! In view of the extensive and thorough nature of the investigations it seems surprising that more prominence has not been given to his findings. In von Pohl's case, it is probable that other professionals were put off as he overstated his case — for von Pohl declared that bad *underground currents* were the cause of every kind of illness! In general, we suspect that the lack of notice taken was largely because scientists and academics could not explain the mechanism satisfactorily, or measure underground currents with any instrument. Therefore, for them, the phenomena did not exist! This attitude still exists to a significant degree, but many professionals are now taking the matter seriously, even if they don't understand it.

Terminology

One of the problems in any discussion of these matters is in the terminology. Von Pohl referred to 'underground currents'. Other words often used for the same effect by various dowsers are: black streams, underground water, ley line, geopathic stress and earth energy: there may be others. Underground water is often thought to be the cause of a problem. This may or may not be the case, depending on the quality of the energy in any water. There is often confusion here, probably for historical reasons. Dowsing was usually thought of only as a method of finding water as this was the only application to survive church censorship. Thus, if a dowser got a reaction from his instrument in places where people suffered bad health, then it must be due to the water because that was all dowsers were expected to find. The term *ley line* is now generally used to describe straight lines linking sacred sites, usually visible across the landscape. Energy lines, whether or not they are associated with sacred site alignments, are usually referred to by dowsers as *energy leys*. The terminology is still subject to change.

We have come to name sacred sites as *thin places*. A friend told us that when he was travelling to Iona, (an island holy to St Columba, who brought Christianity to Scotland), he stopped for fuel at a remote garage on the Isle of Mull. When he told the man filling his car where he was going, the man's eyes went misty and he said, 'Och aye, that's a thin place; there's not much between thee and the Lord up there'. Sure enough, the magical energies of Iona captivated us too in due course, and we recognised that same magic at other sacred sites, although some of the most popular ones are now so commercialised and trampled on it is less easy to sense anything. Significant reactions are more likely to be felt in old churches off the beaten track, which were built on crossings of energy leys. Kilpeck church, in Ann's native Herefordshire, is a favourite.

Perhaps an analogy would be helpful here. Think of the major energy leys as being like the lines of the national grid — the wires conducting electricity at high voltage all over the country. We are not talking about electricity as such, but we see the energy leys we are treating as stepped-down versions of the major leys. They have been through distribution transformers, split and reduced in size and 'voltage' by a system of circles, stones and other markers, until they are domestically useable. Our working hypothesis is that the whole system was positive, i.e. life-enhancing for humans, when it was formed with planet Earth, and ancient peoples recognised and honoured the system with their rituals and edifices. Over millennia the machinations of men have, mostly unconsciously, distorted this system, and caused alterations of both position and polarity. Some healers are looking to restore or re-enhance the system in large areas of landscape; others, like us, are focussing on the needs of inhabitants of individual dwellings, when requested. We all try to do what we can.

There are as many ways of mapping these energies as there are dowsers. One law put forward is that everyone will see these subtle energies differently even if they are learning from the same teacher! Some of the most common mappings are in grids — notably Hartmann grids and Currie grids. Hamish Miller and Paul Broadhurst have dowsed a pair of lines they call Michael and Mary weaving their way right across the country from

Cornwall to Norfolk, touching many sacred sites along the way, as reported in their book (*see* Bibliography and References 5.3). They are pursuing similar findings in Europe for a further volume. Other dowsers find spirals and other shapes. Many dowsers who find energies detrimental to the inhabitants of a place recommend moving house, or moving furniture such as beds where people spend a lot of time. Some market gadgets that protect from the effects of geopathic stress. A few are healing the energies, as we do, so that they are life-enhancing rather than draining. One thing that does matter if healing is to be effective, is that the healer(s) doing the work map out the energies in their own way — then it works. Trying to heal on someone else's mapping is likely to be unsatisfactory, as the map is a personal mind tool through which to navigate and access energies.

The term *geopathic stress* would seem to imply mechanical stress in the earth such as fault lines, for example. Certainly geological fault lines often seem to have a subtle energy effect; but again there seem to be so many energy lines that we doubt that they are all related to earth faults. Our preference is for the term *earth energy*.

In our work we are concerned only with the energies within the subtle environment within houses and workplaces, and their effect on the people who consult us. By this we mean the effects of influences which do not necessarily have a physical, measurable connection, but which are affecting people at subtle levels. Sensitive people, kinesiologists and dowsers, who are sometimes given the title of 'biosensors', can detect them. Some scientific instrumentation is being developed to find these kinds of effects, but is still experimental and relies heavily on the interpretation of the operator. We have learned something about Bicom and Vega machines, and we have had a Best device demonstrated to our healing group. We feel that focussing on the quality of this energy itself is the important factor rather than being worried about the presence of water, geological fault lines, sacred sites or any other features.

Research

Detecting results of geopathic stress has, however, been tested scientifically. Dr Bergsmann, a university consultant in medicine in Vienna, undertook an extensive study to investigate the influence of earth energies on health in 1990 (*see* Bibliography and References 3.3). The Austrian Government funded this research. Dr Bergsmann measured 24 parameters on each of 985 test people; i.e. he tested 24 different kinds of medical investigation on each person — a very extensive programme. He used 3 dowsers to locate places of geopathic stress and neutral places in 8 hospital rooms in various places in Austria. The 24 parameters were tested first, after each subject had stayed 15 minutes in a neutral place. They were then repeated after the subject had stayed 15 minutes in the geopathic stress place, and then again with the subject after 15 minutes in the neutral place. In all, 6,943 investigations were carried out giving over 500,000 data points that were statistically evaluated.

These parameters, or medical tests, included electrical resistance of the skin, circulation system tests such as heartbeat, blood pressure, orthostatic reactions and blood tests. There were muscle reflex and physical tests and, perhaps importantly, neurotransmitter tests including serotonin production.

The results showed 12 of the tests were significantly affected by geopathic stress. In 5 tests some effect was found, and in 6 others there was no effect. This is an exceedingly clear result showing that place can be a very important factor in health. Especially interesting was the highly significant reduction in serotonin levels, which affects sleep patterns. People often report poor sleep when their bed is over a geopathic stress zone, a finding well known to dowsers. This has now been validated by scientific experiment. We understand that Dr Bergsmann is doing more research.

Some years ago dowsers traced some negative earth energies in a village on a small British island, and then asked the local GP to check his records for the number of inhabitants of homes on these lines who had suffered from degenerative diseases. Every house on these black lines had a history of chronic illness and an unusually high number of cancer victims. A doctor might concern himself with environmental health at a physical level, e.g. a sufferer with a lung complaint would be better away from factory and traffic fumes. But anyone seeking to improve their health also needs to attend to the state of the earth energies at their home and place of work.

We are sometimes asked how common are these energy lines that we find. It's not possible to say in overall terms, as we are only approached by people who think there is something wrong at their location. We occasionally have to tell clients that some other cause must be at work as we find no lines, or only positive ones, at their address. Mostly we are finding between one and four energy lines, rarely more, at any given place. Sometimes there is a mixture of positive and negative ones, and this can feel more uncomfortable to the inhabitants than all negative: there is a two-way pull which is very unsettling.

Energies in Water

So far we have only mentioned earth energies, or geopathic stress in the context of health and place. The noted French scientist, Jacques Benveniste, has carried out very interesting research into the subtle nature of water. He was research director at the French National Institute for Medical Research and specialised in the mechanisms of allergy and inflammation. In 1984, while working on hypersensitive (allergic) systems he came upon the so-called, high dilution phenomena. This was picked up by the media and labelled the 'memory of water'. He showed that water has a memory and that information can therefore be stored in it. This is the basis of homoeopathy. To make a homoeopathic remedy, a small amount of the appropriate substance is dissolved in water. This water is shaken (succussed), diluted, shaken, diluted and the process repeated again many times. The final result is virtually pure water as very little, if any, of the originally dissolved substance remains. Nevertheless this water can have powerful curative properties (*see* Bibliography and References 3.11). In fact, the less of the appropriate *substance* there is, the more powerful it is as a homoeopathic remedy.

As is so often the case with people who come up with revolutionary concepts, orthodoxy rejected his ideas. To so many people, water was no more than a chemical combination of hydrogen and oxygen and the very idea of information being stored therein was just preposterous. Although a number of scientists looked into his work and agreed with him, he was forced out of the senior position he held in the government laboratory. He has now set up his own laboratory, supported by industrial and financial investors, and continues his work.

Alan Hall, an innovative scientist, has done some very interesting work looking at water (*see* Bibliography and References 3.6). Water is very significant in all life processes. About eighty per cent of the human body is water, and our lives depend on being able to replenish it regularly. Its importance to the plant kingdom is very obvious. We all know that you must water your plants if they are to flourish, or even to grow at all! Alan concludes that water can contain information that is vital to life processes. This information is held within the arrangement of the microstructure of water. An analogy is the way that information, such as music or video pictures, is contained in the magnetic characteristics of the iron oxide dust deposited on recording tapes. Alan has found that this life-force information within water can be corrupted by outside influences in a similar way that the music can be corrupted on a tape, particularly if it is too near a magnet. One of the main sources of information corruption in water is by the various electromagnetic fields that are constantly growing in their complexity. These fields come from electric power lines, microwave telecommunication links, mobile phones etc. Thus, you can be adversely affected by the information quality of the water piped to your house as much as by its chemical impurity as delivered by the water company and/or by your household filtering system. One way this corruption may occur is when the electric company places a transformer in the street over the water main. Another way may be due to the location of your central heating pump within the plumbing such that the electric field from the motor cuts across a circulation pipe. Thus, the *nasty vibes* are being pumped round and round the house. Our society is unlikely to do away with electricity, telecommunications and all the other technical devices that can degrade water.

We have been following Alan's research for some years and relating it to our own work. There is some overlap, as we often find that if we have transmuted the earth energies at a house then the informational content of the water is no longer a problem. We are all learning more about these matters, but additional research and correlation is required into the relationship between the information held within water (which is nearly always present) and that in the phenomenon we call earth energies.

Other Indications of a Sick House

A further source of subtle pollution can come from equipment in the home: in particular, the domestic electrical wiring. Some people react adversely to this, and also to the emanations from TV sets and computers. Microwave ovens are also a possible problem. If they leak microwaves then this can be harmful, but they are unlikely to be a major problem because they are usually switched on only for a very short time. Perhaps of more concern is the effect they have on food cooked in them. There is evidence that irradiating food with microwaves can destroy the subtle content of the food. This is likely to be most significant if they are used to cook freshly harvested vegetables.

Some research has been done in Switzerland, (*see* Bibliography and References 3.7), on the use of microwave ovens for reheating babies' milk in hospitals. This concluded that the milk was significantly degraded. Manufacturers of microwave ovens took the authors to court in an attempt to have their report suppressed, which makes one suspect that the research was valid! In any case it would seem to correlate with Alan Hall's findings concerning the effect of electromagnetic fields on the information in water. Unfortunately, food technologists and nutritionists do not seem to take into account any subtle component of food. They only look at the physical part.

Any review of the influence of place on health would be incomplete without reference to the possible effects of *presences* — we will deal with these in Chapter 6. There are many influences beyond our normal world as we perceive it with our five senses.

Animals can often indicate energy lines and spots as well as being aware of presences. It appears that bees, ants and also cats thrive in negative places, dogs thrive in positive places; but we have not researched this very thoroughly, just noticed some examples. One woman phoned to ask if we had done the healing on her house that morning. We had, but why did she ask? Her dog had always refused to eat his food in the kitchen, where we had located a negative line. That morning he accepted it happily, and continued to eat in the kitchen thereafter.

Cats are well known for resting in warm places near fires and radiators, and next to warm bodies. But many sit in odd places unconnected with sources of warmth, and these places are often where there are negative energies. We have reports that these pets become disturbed when the lines are healed and take time to settle into the house's new energy patterns. Some clients have sent their house plans with marks showing where their cat sleeps!

If you know what to look for, the presence of energy lines can often be seen from the form of growth of trees with peculiar bends and distortions from their normal shape. Alan Hall told us one of the most interesting cases. He was walking through a wood and noted that many trees had dropped large numbers of twigs. The point of fracture of these twigs was all similar and looked as if they had split round circumferentially more and more until finally the little pip in the centre had parted dropping the twig. He had also noticed that the trees so affected were in a straight line. He followed this line to the edge of the wood and found himself looking at a large satellite dish aimed straight at him across the valley. This dish was part of a major government communications facility. We have also received reports of people being adversely affected by communication dishes pointed at their houses. When the owners are finally persuaded to point their dish in some other direction, they feel better. If they feel worse again it is sometimes found that the dish has been returned to its previous direction on the basis that people have now forgotten about it.

It is not uncommon for the presence of earth energies to be indicated by the shape of the growth of plants and trees. Part of our garden consists of an old orchard. There was a line of four trees which all exhibited similar characteristics. In each case shortly after the tree emerged from the ground the trunk bent over nearly ninety degrees before again growing up vertically. This was very clear in the first tree but was less marked in the last in the line. Dowsing indicated an earth energy line running under the points where the trunks were vertical. It was as though the trees felt that they had been planted in the wrong place and had tried to grow to where they really wanted to be! Some of these trees also had odd knobbly lumps and burls on their trunks and branches. This feature is also often a sign that growth is being influenced by earth energies. Sadly, three of these four old trees have now succumbed to gales.

Evidence of Effects

Overall there is plenty of evidence that many of these things affect human health. The effects are often very subtle. The modern materialistic scientist does not have instruments to detect these effects and he often finds the data from dowsers inconsistent. Anecdotal evidence and observations from doctors can be very helpful. Dr K. told us:

'I have observed the following from my experience with patients:

'Infant not sleeping well and crying at night; changing bed position stopped the above.

'Lady, forty-three years old, right ovarian cyst, pre-cancerous, became totally well after G.S. from house healed.

'Also, patients with geopathic problems keep relapsing despite treatment once they return to their home — in fact become sicker, and have problems more in the evenings and night.'

The research in Austria reported above should be seen as very significant. We need to keep on observing, and measuring what and when we can, (*see* Chapter 10), until a viable pattern emerges; which is, after all, how every branch of science found its roots. What matters is the beneficial effect on people of working in this way.

Chapter 2

SOME SIGNIFICANT EARLY CASES

It was surprising how soon after learning our skills in healing sick houses we started having enquiries. Nowadays, one might put one's readiness for service in any particular area out on the Internet but twenty years ago that had hardly developed; so, we just put it out on the subtle ethers and there was no need for promotional leaflets or advertising — people in need just found us.

In this chapter we tell stories of healings. The practicalities are described in Chapter 5.

Our early efforts were as taught by Bruce MacManaway, and then developed further as we learned more from our own experience. Ann had been working as a kind of apprentice with Bruce, a healer from Scotland, in the 1970s. It was not until the summer school in 1979 that he started teaching his method of healing sick houses to his student group. Ann was booking in to the second year of his week long training sessions at a hotel in Warwickshire when Roy suddenly announced that he wanted to come too. It was for the development of practising healers (which Roy was not), cost money (which we were short of), and he would have to take leave from his job at short notice (he would just tell them he wouldn't be in next week).

'Perhaps Bruce will not accept you,' Ann warned. But Bruce dowsed for Roy's suitability and we attended the event together. ... It was one of those 'meant to be' occasions.

Bruce was teaching his methods of healing people through dowsing and pressures on the spine and other gentle man-oeuvres. He was also teaching about the importance of *ley lines* or *earth energies*, in relationship to health. He showed us his method of detection by dowsing and how to alter the quality of these energies by driving metal poles into exactly the right place in the ground. To Roy's surprise and pleasure it seemed that he could do this with great accuracy. Thus he had finally found out why he had been shown how to dowse some years earlier.

What was next? Well, people of whom we had never heard, started to approach us, saying, 'We hear you can correct black streams under houses. We think we are being affected, so would you please come and sort them out for us?' They seemed to benefit from our efforts and they told others. More and more requests came in. Roy was still in full-time employment and Ann was working too, so the number of cases we could deal with was limited and sometimes people had to wait a bit before we could attend to them.

A House in Middle England

A plea for help arrived from a family in Buckinghamshire. A woman in her fifties had been suffering from depression. She improved when cared for in hospital but went downhill again when she went home, and this pattern had been going on for five years or so. She had lived in the house for twenty-five years, and found it a happy house for bringing up her family, so what was wrong with it? They sent us a map of the place.

We dowsed for the earth energies affecting it. We found two negative lines running through, which we marked on the map. On the next available Saturday we drove to her home, complete with dowsing tools and a bootful of lengths of strong angle iron, hacksaw and sledgehammer. We were on a mission to adjust the energies using a kind of earth acupuncture.

After dowsing around her garden, we plotted the lines and located exactly where their centres were on the ground. We found spots on these centre lines at the edges of the garden, in flower-beds where we would not damage anything by hammering in stakes. Then we ascertained, again by dowsing, how long the stakes should be; it could be anything from a few inches to

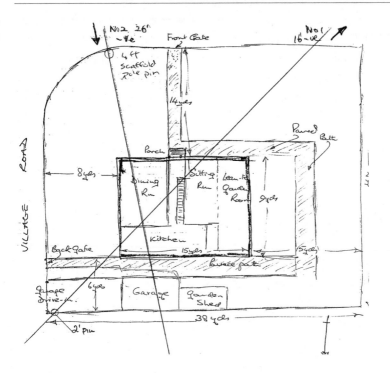

Figure 2.1 — Map of a House in Buckinghamshire Showing Negative Lines

four or five feet, and they had to be inserted into the ground until they had completely disappeared. We found that the required length was not necessarily the same on the day of the *pinning* as it was a few days before when working on the map at home, so we sawed them to size on-site. Then, with due intent, we hammered them into the selected spots on the edge of the property. One line was 26 feet wide, the other 16 feet, so there wasn't much of the house remaining unaffected. The centres of the lines crossed near the kitchen, so sensitive people would most likely be drained at subtle levels if they spent time there.

It turned out that the woman's troubles had started as she went into the menopause, a likely time for increased sensitivity when hormone balances are unstable. We thought that her depression might not have taken hold if she had had only the menopause to deal with, but negative earth energies as well had tipped her over the edge.

On the earth energies course with Bruce MacManaway we were interested in his concept that these energy lines were connected with the network of ley lines criss-crossing the whole country, so we had mapped an extension of the larger line on an ordnance survey map to see where it came from.

We found its origin in a hilltop site where a number of pathways converged, and thought it was likely that this was originally a sacred site. Such places were used for maypole dancing and other rituals to enhance the energies in the countryside, and are often referred to as *trendles*. There might have been a stone or tree circle there, but when we visited the site there was no sign of these, only the trackways radiating from it. Tracing the line back toward the house we had just healed, we found it *positive* until it crossed an area at the beginning of the bypass road around the local town, and then changed to *negative* until it reached the house. We explored this on the ground and found there had been major earthworks to construct the slip road in to this bypass. This is just the kind of thing that Bruce told us changes the polarity of lines, which have been positive and helpful to people for millennia. On our return home we phoned the family we had just visited and asked when the bypass had been built. 'Between five and six years ago,' they said, 'shortly before Mother became ill.' Since that time we have found a great many examples of lines changing to negative polarity where the earth has been considerably disturbed. Active quarries are a nightmare in this respect, as blasting happens periodically, and any healing work on the energies is reversed again.

We were very happy to hear that this woman, whose home we healed, stayed well from that time onwards and did not have to return to hospital. Some years later she moved away, still well.

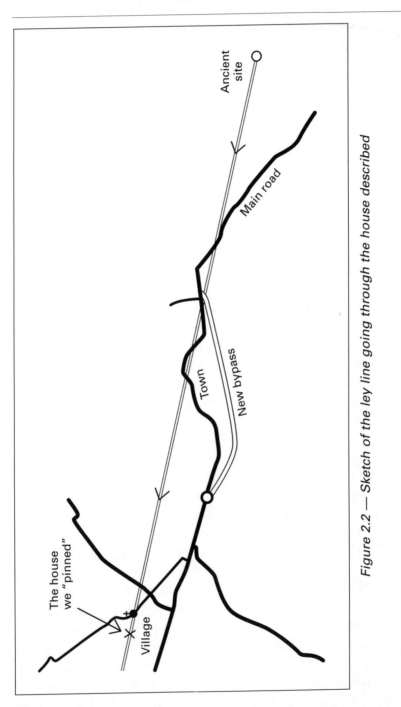

Figure 2.2 — Sketch of the ley line going through the house described

A VIP Mansion

Another early case was an impressive and prestigious house in government ownership. The occupants changed every three years and there were a large number of functions held there, hosting important guests. There had been sightings of ghosts, 'things going bump in the night' and some poltergeist activity. The lady of the house became alarmed, especially when she realised that there had been several cases of cancer and serious illness among previous incumbents and their families. A friend of hers had been on one of Bruce's courses with us, and since we lived nearby, suggested she contact us.

Again we obtained a map, dowsed to plot the lines, and then visited. In the course of dowsing on-site it became apparent that one energy line was negative through the house, but positive in the far flowerbed where we might have driven our stake. This was something new! The line had changed to negative some-where along the way. We dowsed to find where this had hap-pened, as this would be the place to *pin* it. Our elder daughter, then in her late teens, had come with us on this expedition as she was home for the weekend, and had been chatting with the lady. She knew nothing of this healing work then, and had just come along for the ride. Without knowing what we had found, she walked down the line from the flowerbed toward the house, and stopped dead in her tracks shuddering and exclaiming, 'It turns into black treacle here'. Not everyone needs to use dows-ing tools!

The gentleman resident in the house had been studying its journal. Each incumbent had recorded repairs and renovations and events relevant to the care of the house over many years. He found that about twelve years previously a tree surgeon had been called in to give an opinion on one of the two magnificent cedar trees on the lawn. They were several hundred years old and a significant feature of the extensive gardens. One of them at that time was distinctly unwell, and the tree surgeon had advised it be felled — i.e. he had condemned it. Later that day the tree surgeon had a fatal heart attack, and the tree never was cut down. The place where he may well have stood to make his condemning statement was in the middle of the lawn where we had found the energy line had changed to negative. We suggest that the tree took the life-force of the man, and this exchange turned the line to negative at that spot.

Certainly the tree looked very well when we were there, far from being in a state to be condemned. We drove our stake in that spot, making sure it ended well below the surface out of the way of mowing attention to the immaculate lawn! We drove another stake elsewhere in the garden to heal the other line: the lady said she felt very shocked as we did it: 'It was like piercing a mandrake through the heart,' she said. All the anomalies in the house ceased and our clients completed their tenure of the house in peace. We have kept in touch with them over the years, dowsing, and where necessary healing, the various houses they have occupied.

A House Near a Crossroads

Another interesting example in those early days was a house very near to our previous home in Surrey. The man living there came to see Ann professionally for tuition in relaxation and some spiritual healing for his frequent migraines. At some stage he noted that the migraines never happened when he was away from home, so Ann dared to mention that this might be due to negative earth energies at his house. In due course we visited his home and pinned the lines. He noticed that one was coming from a house where a pop group lived, taking drugs and creating a lot of noise nuisance etc. So, at his request, we traced the line across a lane on the other side of this house and found it positive. It seems that in this case a line was *turned negative* directly due to the behaviour of these inhabitants.

Further on along the line, downstream as it were, was a road junction where five roads met, and several accidents had happened there. One of the roads had been a driveway to a large house, now turned into a housing estate. Two magnificent, (if you like that sort of thing!), Victorian brick pillars flanked this driveway, topped with spheres of brick construction, and these were right on the energy line. These pillars had been damaged a number of times by vehicles, although there was plenty of room to pass between. Soon after we healed this line a local bricklayer made it the final job of his working life to rebuild the pillars, complete with spherical finials. A plaque was unveiled marking this event, with pictures in the local paper. The general opinion was that they would not last long judging by previous experience. But they are still there! No-one else bumped into them now that the line through them was positive. In the several years that we remained living nearby, there were no more accidents at that crossroads. It made us wonder how many road — and other — accidents might be at least partly caused by being on negative earth energy lines. The relaxed hands of a driver on the steering wheel are not unlike the hands of a dowser on his rods: if they twitch when crossing a line, what happens to the vehicle?

Two London Houses

Another significant step forward happened when a friend who was fighting secondary cancer, (and won, she is still with us eighteen years on!), asked us to dowse her London house. There was a negative line which needed healing, but we could not put an iron stake in the required place because there was a concrete floor to her utility area right up to the wall of the neighbour's house. *Upstairs* (*see* Chapter 5) was giving us another lesson, it seemed. What were we supposed to learn? After a considerable amount of head scratching and dowsing, we asked the friend to find a piece of metal exactly the right length, and place it horizontally in exactly the right place next to the neighbour's wall. Our dowsing responded that it had done the job of healing her negative line. The next time we visited we observed a piece of metal strip used for supporting shelf brackets tucked comfortably behind her vegetable rack. As far as we know it is still there!

As if to emphasise the point, a week or two later came another request from London friends, this time in a third-floor penthouse flat, with no access to the ground. The lady was keen for us to do our stuff, the man was a bit sceptical, but willing for us to try: he had been sleeping badly. So again we offered the DIY solution: a length of copper pipe **exactly** the right length (by dowsing) in **exactly** the right place; lying on the floor with its centre on the centre of the line against the wall of the loo on the mezzanine floor, just before entering their flat. A crystal was also to be positioned on the floor in one of the rooms to connect the healing with the top floor. Bless them, they did as we suggested! We noticed an improvement in the subtle atmosphere next time we visited, and then received the man's report:

'These things are so subjective; could it be that the weather got cooler just as the copper rod was put in? Or that my work stress got less? Or Pluto got off my Ascendant degree? Or whatever? I don't know, but sceptical as I am, there does seem to be a difference! I am sleeping better/deeper and don't wake so often. Now, of course, I was not aware really of being troubled, well not much and only sporadically. So it was phasic for me anyway. But as I say, there does seem to be a difference, and it is significant, and I am both delighted, grateful and happily surprised. Bless you and thank you both.'

Beginning to Heal Remotely

Then, a little later, Roy was in Canada on a business trip. He got talking about dowsing with someone at an evening gathering and was asked to dowse her house. As there was healing to be done, he was invited along on the following Sunday morning to her place on the outskirts of Vancouver, taking his bemused colleague with him. He found the house was built on solid rock, so there was no way he could hammer in a stake in the standard MacManaway fashion. So he continued his dowsing, and found that a copper pipe laid along a step in the garden, like a stair rod, would be appropriate. At this point Roy asked his hostess to provide him with a phone, and called Ann in Surrey to double-check his findings. We always do this work together, and he saw no reason why he should do without her evaluation just because she was on the other side of the world! The healing worked fine.

So it seemed we could get away without the sledge-hammering part of the job, and both of us didn't necessarily have to be present when the artefact was placed in or on the ground to trigger the healing reaction.

A number of cases later we were asked to dowse an impressive manor house a long way from home. We would not be able to visit for some weeks due to pressure of work and a planned holiday. These people sounded pretty desperate: their son, aged twenty-one, was going off the rails; and it was noted that he was using the same bedroom in which his grandmother was sleeping when she went blind. A stream ran in a culvert under the house, including the room in question. On this occasion we found, through dowsing their map, that this negative energy line did relate to underground water, and another negative line crossed it under the suspect room.

The need for healing was urgent, as the son was at risk of being diagnosed schizophrenic. Well, we were used to sending distant healing to people, why not to a house? So we focussed on the map, and the owner's letter, and we called on the Christ Spirit to help, and it worked. Thereafter, we started to save time, energy and petrol by doing the healing as well as the dowsing work on various jobs using maps and letters to focus upon. Perhaps we didn't always need to visit the location in person. At first we thought it would be just a *first aid* job to help the people until we could get there and hammer in the necessary iron stakes. But no, the places stayed healed, and so we continued our practice in this form. The focussed intent of our minds became just as effective as the physical effort of hammering in a metal stake. However, we do suggest that it was important for us to learn these skills by working on the actual ground, and that it is best for beginners to get initial experience visiting and hammering if possible.

Nowadays we only very rarely go to a house to facilitate a healing. Occasionally an owner insists, and until we started

teaching more dowsers/healers how to do it, we have occasionally complied. Such expeditions are always an adventure, sometimes exhausting, with much pleasure and amusement as well as
learning situations. On 8 August 1988, (8.8.88), we were persuaded to go to a house not far from home, and promised dinner when we had done the job. When we arrived the hostess
revealed that she had invited eight people to dinner and that
they were all interested in what we were doing. We had an audience and were obliged to sing for our supper! It is not easy to
be focussed enough for accurate dowsing, let alone operate in a
healing mode, with several hungry guests, sherry glasses in
hand, asking innumerable questions and needing to be protected from any adverse effects (*see* Chapter 9).

Healing a Sick Stable

On another occasion a fearsome Somerset farmer's wife of ample
proportions insisted that we visited in person to heal two lines
running through the stable of her prize show horse. Here was a
huge and beautiful beast who was kicking so uncontrollably that
she had padded his stable with straw bales: we were glad he was
shut in! The farmer, literally sucking a straw and leaning over the
gate as in a Giles cartoon, watched us with wry amusement. Two
sons with biceps like weightlifting champions offered to saw our
two stakes to the right length, and did it in a flash. It took no
time at all for them to hammer them into the ground — all four
and three feet of metal respectively. We had enthusiastic reports
of the stallion's prowess thereafter, and he no longer kicked his
stable to pieces.

Although such expeditions are very interesting and rewarding, we could not possibly execute the volume of work we now
undertake if we went physically to each one. And we are finding that more and more people are not bothered by the fact that
we never go to their houses to heal them; doing such things at
a distance is becoming more acceptable.

We have so many stories like this, and will be presenting
some more recent ones written by the clients themselves in

Chapter 7. The important thing for us is that we learned more about the nature of these harmful energies and how to heal them, by experiencing cases such as those described. This process of learning continues and expands, nearly twenty years on, and we hope that never stops. There is a saying that you are old when you finish learning!

Chapter 3

BRIDGES BETWEEN
SUBTLE AND PHYSICAL

In order to do this work we have to access intuition in a very precise way. How do we do this? Our culture has brought us up to believe in what has been proved, and to distrust or generally give lower status to anything which does not fit into a framework of A + B = C. All the ramifications of that way of approaching the world are generally known as the scientific method.

Edward de Bono, in the 1960s, described the difference between vertical thinking and lateral thinking. Vertical thinking involves proving something, and then putting it alongside another proved something. It is then possible to deduce something further, and put it on top of the first two, like an overlapping building block.

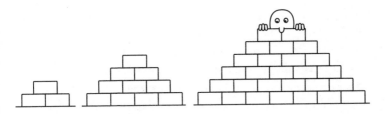

Figure 3.1 — Illustration of the Process of Vertical Thinking

This process can continue until you have a brick wall in front of you, with everything neatly proved and accepted as truth. It's quite possible for the wall to become so high and complicated that you cannot see over it, let alone through or round it!

Lateral thinking is like making up a jigsaw puzzle with an infinite number of pieces, and no helping picture on the box. It's the way small children form their view of the world, long before they can use words. They observe what is going on, and gradually make connections, such as, 'When they sit me in my high chair I am likely to get food' or 'If they put my coat on, we are probably going out'. They are putting pieces of the jigsaw together, and gradually there will be more and more little pictures, which at some stage can be connected up with each other and make up the whole. Except that the jigsaw of life is never finished, and what we have in our minds at any one time is a collection of hypotheses that serve for now. Some hypotheses may be put aside very quickly because they don't fit other pieces of the puzzle, even if they are proved correct: they seem as if they come from another puzzle. Some may stay on the table and last a lifetime because they are central to our individual world picture. Lateral thinking is vital to dowsing and healing work, and the only proof is that it works — i.e. individuals observe and judge the results and find where these fit into their own jigsaw, as they have formed it so far.

Such concepts of our thinking processes could be seen as masculine and feminine. The psychologist Carl Jung's key principle of the *Anima* and the *Animus* is relevant here. He proposed that whatever gender our physical bodies demonstrate, we all have both masculine and feminine components at the psychological level. He called the feminine in the male the Anima, and the masculine in the female the Animus, and worked on the premise that in order to become more whole — 'individuated' was his term — we need to become aware of and embrace our other half. Ann finds this most appropriate in her psychotherapy work. The beautiful symbol below illustrates Jung's point.

We certainly notice in the groups we teach that men and woman can be (but are certainly not always) polarised. Many men are more comfortable and have been trained more rigorously in vertical thinking, so they need help with using the lateral thinking facility. Women are more likely to be busy making

Figure 3.2 — The Yin/Yang symbol illustrating Jung's theory.

their jigsaws and are sometimes insufficiently logical to construct their questioning clearly, which is vital for effective dowsing. So, doing this work is not only fruitful in terms of results obtained, it also encourages the practitioner in his or her path toward wholeness. Some of the trends in our society are toward women becoming experts in science or engineering, and men becoming carers and healers. In the past, lateral thinking men or women have been given less status and financial reward than vertical thinkers unless they became famous or obviously successful.

Further, and very broadly, we can use the idea that different sides of the brain are used for the different thinking functions. The left side of the brain runs the right side of the body at a physical level. In work using symbology, e.g. dream interpretation, right-sided experiences are seen to be influenced by the masculine. At a mental level the left brain does the logical, brick-building thinking. The right side of the brain runs the left side of the body, the feminine side, at a physical level; on a mental level it thinks laterally and accesses the intuition.

Dowsing involves both, and in particular needs an ability to change from one to the other smoothly and easily, like clicking a switch. There is a physical part of the brain called the corpus callosum, which is the link between the right and left sections of the brain, designed for this purpose, so we are not suggesting the impossible!

The term *gnowing* has been coined for the result of this combination of brain function. In pioneering work of this kind terminology is still developing and is not yet fixed: this does have advantages, however, in allowing further developments without undue restriction.

Levels of Awareness

Here is a diagram to aid understanding about what is happening within ourselves when this type of work is being done:

Here are seven levels of human awareness. It's just one map

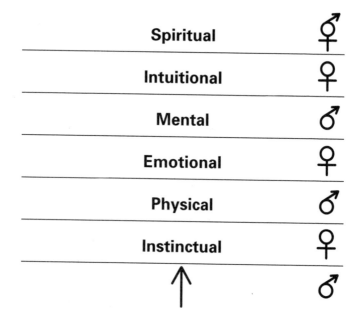

Figure 3.3 — The Levels of Human Awareness

of many useful ones, but the number seven comes up frequently in various philosophies about the human condition. Note that we have marked the masculine and feminine oriented level in the right column. The Mars glyph (♂) represents masculine; it is used to denote male in medical records and is also the astrological glyph for the planet Mars, the masculine God of the Romans (Aries for the Greeks). The Venus glyph (♀) represents the feminine, female in medical records, and the astrological glyph for Venus, the feminine Goddess. When concerned with dowsing, we are looking to use both the mental level, which is on the masculine side, and intuition, on the feminine side, as described above.

From the masculine point of view, differentiation between instinctive, emotional and intuitive levels is difficult, and this can feel threatening. The emotional level relates to having feelings about something, and needs to be transcended when dowsing. If you are concerned for your screaming child in the middle of the night, you would be far too involved to dowse for a homoeopathic remedy, for instance, as you would feel the need to be checking for symptoms of serious disease and wondering whether to call the doctor. You would be too emotionally involved to access your detached intuition and get a clear picture of what is needed. We all have masses of emotional concerns tucked away in the pigeonholes of our brains, and if these surface while dowsing they cloud the issue. We quote from Dr Christine Page:

'Intuition has been defined as "intellect without fear" and as "the immediate grasp of the truth as it essentially exists". It is available to everyone, helping each to walk with steady intent whilst maintaining clear vision. Yet despite conscious awareness of such insight, many fail to act on its advice, which can appear illogical, selfish or out of tune with society. It is only afterwards that we regret not listening to its inner guidance. Other people believe that they are intuitive when tapping into their gut feelings, not recognising that these sensations are strongly allied to past emotional memories which may no longer be appropriate or reliable.'

To trust your intuition, and therefore the dowsing, which is demonstrating it, you need to be detached from what you feel about the situation under consideration. Many people do not differentiate between intuition and emotion. We were giving a talk some time ago, and a distinguished neuropsychiatrist in the audience remarked that he saw Roy as doing the logical/mental part of our work (which was seen as valuable), and Ann doing the emotional part. She felt quite emotional (angry!) about his remark, as she had spent much time and effort trying to differentiate and use only the intuitive level. He said he didn't know the difference! We suspect it was all lumped together as *feminine* stuff to him! Emotions are absolutely fine in their place, though we are often trained to deny and hide them in our British way, but they are inappropriate to dowsing work and need to be expressed in other more appropriate situations.

The instinctive level is interesting in this context. The term instinct is an anathema to mainstream psychology, definitions being difficult and imprecise. Our hypothesis so far puts it in the realm of the animal awareness in us humans. Our understanding is that we are made physically very much on the same pattern as animals, but we have the extra attributes which make us humans. Along with the animals, we have something in us which strives for survival of the individual and of the species. So we see to it that we get food, shelter if necessary, and can procreate and protect our young. In the field of dowsing in general this is rarely relevant, yet when it comes to earth energies and geopathic aspects of our environment, we often find animals are very wise in ways which we have forgotten or overlaid in our so-called civilised existence. Some animals, such as dogs, avoid negative or draining energies; cats love them, and often rest on sink spots or lines which would be detrimental to humans. The latter have a reputation for taking on negative vibrations on behalf of their owners or homes, and earthing them out of the way, the so-called 'witch's cat syndrome'. We probably need to make use of our instinctive faculties to a certain extent when assessing geopathic stress, but not overmuch lest we are damaged in the process. (*See* Protection in Chapter 9.)

Brain Activity

The diagram below illustrates a scale of brain activity using concepts learned from Maxwell Cade and Geoffrey Blundell.

Max was one of the leading experts on mental states in the 1970s and 1980s — his book with Nona Coxhead is called *The Awakened Mind*, (*see* Bibliography and References 8.2). Geoffrey had devised the Mind Mirror, which measures, on a continuous basis, the electrical activity in the brain while people were doing

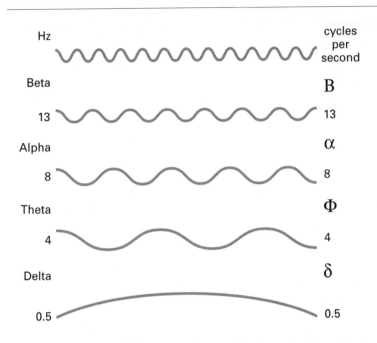

Figure 3.4 — The Scale of Brain Activity According to Cade and Blundell

different types of things with their minds. This sophisticated invention was a development of an instrument which might be used if you went to hospital after suffering a bump on the head. The medics would attach electrodes to your scalp (not uncomfortable, just sticky afterwards!) and obtain a read-out of what' the electrical impulses between the cells in your brain were doing — just to check that things hadn't been damaged inside your skull. It became clear that dowsers were switching between the Beta range of brainwaves, i.e. active, logical, vertical thinking; and the Alpha range, a quieter, receptive, intuitive lateral-thinking state. The rate of electrical activity dropped across the 13 Hz (cycles per second) divide, and back up again. Healers were able to operate in the Theta range as well, and we will come back to that later. If your brainwaves are totally in the Delta range you are in a coma, but some tests with the Mind Mirror showed dowsers with Delta activity in the right brain at the same time as Beta activity in the left. It appears that dowsing requires us to stretch our brains across the full range.

One current, long-held hypothesis is that as brain wave frequency reduces, its owner is less connected with the physical and logical world, and more with the intuitive and spiritual world. We could, but won't, get into theories about near death experiences on this basis. Science is slow to take much interest in paranormal phenomena. One reason is that such matters are not usually amenable to neat, controlled (in scientific terms), repeatable experiments in a laboratory. The other is that most of the activities cannot be measured. There is no earth energy meter for instance, unless you count a dowser, sometimes called a 'biosensor'! And if you do, the results are usually inconsistent and not always repeatable. Thus, scientists who try to venture into this field soon find that their colleagues do not perceive them as good scientists, which is bad for their careers. However, for those readers who may require some sort of a concept of the framework within which the paranormal may be accommodated along with the physical, we recommend *The Vortex* by David Ash and Peter Hewitt (*see* Bibliography and References 3.2).

Energy and Matter

'Matter being formed out of vortices of energy' is a concept that has been handed down from ancient times in Yogi training. In outline, Ash and Hewitt suggest that a fresh look be taken now at the vortex theory of matter put forward by Sir William Thomson (later Lord Kelvin) in the latter part of the nineteenth century. In this theory Sir William put forward the idea that matter was composed of vortices of energy which had the appearance of solid particles, rather than the then current theory of matter being made of very small indivisible solid particles. Most of the leading scientists of the day supported his theory. Nevertheless, the particulate theory was adopted as the basis of matter by the early part of the twentieth century. Later it was found that the atom was not the smallest particle but that it was made up of electrons and other particles, or charges, in orbit.

The vortex theory held that the elemental particle was a vortex of pure energy in which the underlying movement occurs at the speed of light. In other words, matter in our physical universe is made of energy moving at the speed of light. This is consistent with Einstein's theory, which holds that the limitation for us is the speed of light and that at speeds approaching this, time and space undergo fundamental changes. Thus, the speed of light determines the limit of the physical universe, or the boundary of our material world.

However, there does not seem to be any reason to suppose that there are not energies moving at speeds higher than the speed of light. In such a universe, matter could still be formed on the basis of the vortex. But this matter would not be perceptible from our universe. Beings in this higher speed universe would appear to themselves to be existing in a material sense similar to our own, but different laws of physics may apply, although they might be able to perceive our lower speed universe (and possibly have difficulty in understanding its limitations!).

Some of the information channelled from discarnates, souls of people who have left their bodies, would seem to support such a theory. It follows that movement between universes, or states of being, is to do with manipulation of the speed of movement of the formative energy. It is interesting that in some literature there is reference to matter being made of slow light!

It seems likely that the phenomena of resonance may be used to connect between some of these states of being. It is shown that a singer can shatter a wine glass if exactly the right note is sounded. The glass will have its own note when rung. If you hit it too hard it will break. The singer sounds a note that is either this note or a multiple in terms of its frequency, which causes the glass to vibrate in sympathy. By continuing the excitation caused by the singer's note, thus increasing the amplitude of the vibration, the glass will shatter as the vibration becomes too much for the strength of the material.

Similarly in a musical instrument such as a piano, one finds that strings other than the one struck will vibrate. For instance, if a note C is struck it will be found that the string for the C in the next octave will also vibrate in sympathy. This is because the notes in one octave are direct multiples, in terms of their frequency, of the same notes in other octaves. This is the resonance effect whereby one object will vibrate in sympathy with another object if in tune. And these effects not only occur at the same frequency, but also at exact multiples of that frequency.

These examples show how one level can affect another level. So it seems possible that we can relate to some of these other states of existence via the resonance effect if we are able to tune ourselves to an appropriate frequency. How to achieve this state of attunement is difficult to describe in a clear descriptive way; but healers and sensitives are doing it regularly. The most important step is to accept the possibility. For Roy, the logical engineer, it was finding that he could dowse in his late forties that convinced him he had the ability to become attuned, and that this had been latent and dormant all along!

You, the reader, may not care for these concepts and think it's all a load of rubbish. Perhaps they are, but they are interesting thoughts that are worth keeping in mind when becoming further involved in some of these so-called paranormal occurrences. To a large extent we are living with a collection of hypotheses, because the kind of proof science requires cannot accommodate these dimensions of human awareness. We have to rely on gnowing rather than knowing, and put the pieces of our own personal jigsaws of life experience together as best we may.

There is a whole range of impossible activities around staring us in the face. One of the oldest and simplest is dowsing. No-one has proved how that works yet. Then there is remote viewing, which has been developed and used by the military. Sai Baba is probably the most famous demonstrator of manifesting objects out of nothing. Spoon bending is another simple example. Then there are crop circles, a really big phenomenon that could be deemed impossible, but they happen year after year! And of course there are UFOs. Reports have been coming in for years and years, many from completely reliable witnesses. But officially there is no such thing!

A look at some ancient stonework shows enormous, irregularly shaped pieces fitting together perfectly. This process was apparently done without machinery, which would need to be very large indeed to handle the weights involved. So was it done by teleporting? Perhaps the ancients had the secret of free energy devices? There are examples to be seen all over the world. In dowsing and healing we are working with several levels or dimensions of awareness at the same time.

So the limitation to broadening our experience would seem to be our own thought processes and our lack of ability to consider a new paradigm outside the present materialistic basis. This limitation is kept in place by assorted vested interests whether commercial or the reputation of experts.

For many people experiences force them to consider a wider paradigm, and much work is being undertaken by the Scientific and Medical Network (*see* Appendix 1, Resources) to investigate patterns and possibilities. In our own lives Roy noticed that Ann was able to know things intuitively. There were a number of occasions when he phoned home on trips abroad and although these circumstances had no set time or pattern, Ann would answer the phone saying she knew it was him. On one occasion when he phoned from the US she picked the phone up on the first ring. He commented that she must have been at her desk and acted quickly. 'Oh no,' she replied, 'I was out in the garden hanging out the washing.' Roy retorted that she could not have got indoors that fast. 'Well, I knew that you were about to ring, so I put the basket down and went in to the phone. It rang just as I reached it!'

On another occasion Roy was delayed in Paris as bad weather prevented his plane from returning that night. He phoned from the hotel to tell Ann he would be back the next day instead. She asked, 'What happened to you at about 1.30 p.m. today? I felt a very severe bump on my forehead and got a headache that lasted about half an hour.' He told her that he had walked into a glass door, had taken the impact on his forehead and nearly knocked himself out! There were so many coincidences that it was obvious that some subtle process was at work.

The most dramatic example happened to Ann in 1963 and caused her to fear for her sanity. Her father died at her old Herefordshire home. He was aged fifty-seven and had not told us that he had a heart problem. In the depths of that very cold winter Ann was in Surrey bathing our two daughters, then aged nearly four and one-and-a-half, when she perceived in her mind's eye a horrendous scene and passed out cold on the bathroom floor. That evening she attended her painting class — her chief respite from the role of housewife at the time — and tried, unsuccessfully, to paint the scene.

On her return home, Roy was washing up, an unprecedented experience (though he has taken over that chore, with mechanical assistance, since he retired). He sat her down and told her that her father had been trying to thaw the domestic water system and had been found dead across a burning coke brazier. It was her perceived scene!

That night, when she was definitely awake, she saw her Dad sitting on her bed, complete with old tweed jacket with a button missing, and he assured her that his death had been instant, he had not suffered. (A postmortem the next day confirmed a coronary thrombosis.) While she found that very comforting amid all the shock and grief, she was also very worried about her perceptions — they were not 'normal' — and she feared that if she told anyone she would be sent to the local lunatic asylum. Roy treated them as curious rather than pathological when she finally got to tell him. The vicar came with condolences and she tried his reaction, very tentatively. He backed away, but lent her a book, *The Imprisoned Splendour*, by Raynor Johnson (*see* Bibliography and References 2.4), an Australian physicist with theories and stories about other dimensions of awareness. That started us on our journey of understanding.

Theosophy, a scheme of understanding which manifested itself in the late nineteenth century, proposes a hierarchy of levels of awareness very similar to our earlier diagram, and extending it to how consciousness works between lifetimes. A rather large leap, perhaps! Anyway, the concept is that when we leave the physical body we are left with *the rest*; each of which is left in turn, while the consciousness retains a core atom of memory. The next step after the physical is the etheric, or aura, which is sensed by a number of healers and others. After that comes the astral, or emotional body. Presences, or ghosts and similar manifestations, which we deal with in Chapter 6, are seen to be stuck in this area and need help to move on. At the next, the mental level, there is sometimes contact with people still physically incarnate in the form of information which the discarnate soul can now encompass: automatic writing is one way of this being brought through to physical manifestation. Further levels are less likely to reach us directly, but there is acknowledgement that the human being encompasses more awareness in the intuitive and spiritual levels as described before.

Visualisation

Another area of exploration, which has been shown to demonstrate a bridge between subtle and physical, is the new discipline of psychoneuroimmunology (what a mouthful!). This effectively finds and proves the mechanisms for phenomena we have noticed in everyday life, such as psychosomatic disease — that what you feel and think makes a difference to your physical health, through affecting chemical changes in the body.

There has long been the belief that you can change things by thinking positively and appropriately, in the vernacular 'mind over matter'. Carl and Stephanie Simonton in Texas in the 1970s (*see* Bibliography and References 6.7) made a great step forward in this field. Carl was working as a radiologist with cancer patients. One day he was surprised to find that one of his patients was doing much better than he expected, so he asked her what she was doing to achieve her improved state of health. She told him that she spent some time each day sitting quietly, using her imagination, and visualising her cancer shrinking and going away. Stephanie, a psychotherapist, took up this idea, and organised groups of Carl's patients to work on themselves in a similar fashion. The results were very encouraging, and this system of visualisation is now an important tool in the approaches offered to cancer patients seeking alternative ways of helping themselves whilst receiving medical treatment.

What is this visualisation? It is inner work, using the power of the right brain to influence what is happening in the body. It is easily confused with relaxation and meditation techniques, especially as these are often taught to people in the same context. Relaxation is about releasing tension from the physical body, and techniques for this have been taught for fifty years or more on the basis of work by such pioneers as Jane Madders and Laura Mitchell. It is a desirable precursor to meditation and visualisation, because the last two work better if the body is less tense. Ways of engaging in meditation are many and varied, unique to the individual, but the object is to quieten the mind into a passive state. In the field of self-help in cancer it was written about and taught by retired psychiatrist Dr Ainslie Meares in Australia (*see* Bibliography and References 6.6).

Visualisation, by contrast, is an active state of mind. The person devises a scenario, perhaps with the help of a therapist versed in these matters, in which they see the cancer process leaving, diminishing, being disposed of, and the individual being in blooming good health. All this is done with the help of pictorial images, which is why the word visual is used. In fact, there is no need to see or picture anything, just to know that the process you have devised is there present, happening as if real. Some people have very vivid visual imaginations, which is fine for them, but others feel discouraged because they haven't: there is no need for this, any kind of sensing will do fine.

Visualisation is a form of self-healing. It can be extended into helping others in a way that many would call prayer. If you imagine someone is well and healthy, and ask your healing source for that visualisation to become manifest, it works in a similar way. A recent lecture by Dr Peter Fenwick gave details of some scientific research projects, which had demonstrated the efficacy of praying for people, which he equated with healing. William Harris, of St Luke's Hospital in Kansas City, Missouri, US, who studied patients who came into the coronary care unit, conducted one of these. He found that the 466 patients in the group who were prayed for had significantly better outcomes than the 524 patients who received no prayer (unbeknown to any of them). The prayed-for group recovered more quickly and experienced less pain.

There is a huge number of discoveries emerging in this field of links and connections, bridges between subtle awareness and physical experience, some of them scientifically explored and known, many of them still in the area of human gnowing.

Chapter 4

DOWSING AS DETECTOR AND DIAGNOSTIC TOOL

In this chapter we start by looking at ways of explaining dowsing and then describe its practice. If you would like to' run through a dowsing lesson, look in Chapter 8.

What is dowsing? We would describe it as a non-intellectual information acquisition process. Our usual way of acquiring information is to build it up from a series of facts from which other facts can be deduced, as explored in the previous chapter. This process can be continued at great length and the solution to very complex questions can be obtained. It is the basis of the scientific, or *bottom-up* method of information gathering, the deductive process.

The other possibility is to pose the question (left brain) and receive, or recognise, the answer with no intermediate process, the 'top-down' method. Dowsing operates in this way. Of course, the obvious question is from where does the information come? Many of us tend not to believe anything unless we can understand the process or mechanism employed. This is one of the problems with scientific investigations into dowsing because a different paradigm is required.

We do not claim to know exactly how dowsing works. We do gnow that it does. We also know that considerable care and discrimination is required if it is to be an effective tool. So we will put forward some ideas for your consideration. Firstly, we are quite sure that it is not a case of our picking up some sort of emanation from, say, water. On the face of it this does not seem to be unreasonable. A dowser walks across a field with his rods and they move when he passes over water. So the assumption is that he must picking up some invisible influence at that spot due to the presence of the water. Yes, but if the dowser can locate the water when he is miles away and pinpoint the location on a map, that theory is not tenable. Similarly, some dowsers can locate breaks in electric transmission systems from maps and direct the repair crews to the appropriate spot. There are countless other examples of dowsers being able to detect things at considerable distances.

Psychological Considerations

How does the human psyche achieve this? Let us look at it in terms of transpersonal psychology, first mooted by Assagioli (*see* Bibliography and References 8.1) in the 1960s. He demonstrated his theory with the egg diagram as shown below:

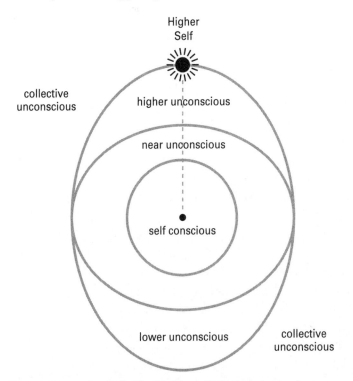

Figure 4.1 — Assagioli's Theory of Transpersonal Psychology

The spot in the centre represents the centre of the personality, the I, the little self, the place from which we are looking out into the world at any given moment. Immediately around it is the area we are conscious of right now. Beyond that is an area of our unconscious that is near the surface, available quite easily via associations and reminders (near unconscious). Then the deeper layers of the unconscious were divided into higher and lower sections, and these are more accessible through dreams and visualisation practices making use of right brain intuitive function, but still belonging to the individual. The link with the spiritual level of that individual was via the Higher Self, or Soul might be a more familiar term, which operated all round the periphery of the egg. Beyond the egg is the collective unconscious, shared by everybody. In this area it is possible for us to find anything we need to know. Perhaps that is what we are tapping into when we dowse?

In considering possible ways in which dowsing works we have to look at the nature of the human being beyond not only our physical bodies, but also beyond the individual psyche. Most religions incorporate the concept of a Super Spirit, God, Goddess or Creator by whatever name may be used. They also teach that there is an aspect of us that continues after death of the physical body. There has been a vast amount of research into past lives and near death experiences which supports these views (*see* Bibliography and References, Section 2). We think that our non-physical component exists in some other state that is not normally accessible to us as physical beings, but is very closely linked to us. In fact it is vital that it is linked as otherwise our body fails to function, 'His spirit has left — he is dead'. This concept leads to the idea that our memories may not be stored in our physical brain, but in this spirit component. This is not to say that memories are not accessed through the brain. We think the brain may be like a radio receiver in that it links to one's own spirit as demonstrated in the egg diagram, and retrieves memories as required. It is no good trying to find the music inside the radio receiver, it is somewhere else, i.e. in the programme being broadcast.

Information Selection

If we had complete access to all information available to the spirit at all times, the results would be overwhelming. Thus, limiters are put into the system for our protection. Dowsing is a way of bypassing some of these limiters and hence accessing information from another level of our being. This other level of our being is not constrained by time and space as we are in our physical body. So it could, for instance, travel to a house needing healing, look over the fence and see the energies affecting it, then come back and report to the dowser. Another way of looking at it is to conceive of a vast library in the sky, which some would call the akashic record. The Internet is similar to this, but in a physical form! Dowsers are allowed access to various sections, according to their speciality. This would account for some, like us, being able to dowse for healing purposes, but hopeless at finding lost objects. There are specialists in the use of dowsing just as in any other skill.

Consider any sort of measuring or recording instrument. It must have parts of itself that are in two separate systems, but the parts must be connected in some way. For instance, a voltmeter, as shown below:

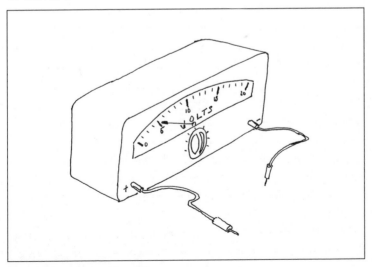

Figure 4.2 — A Voltmeter

The voltmeter has a coil in the electric part and a spring and pointer in the mechanical part. The two parts are connected via magnetic effects induced by the electric current being measured. The coil detects the electricity while the pointer moves to tell us the voltage. We cannot directly determine the voltage of the electricity, however, our eye can see and interpret the movement of the pointer. There are many other examples of devices using two different systems. A piezoelectric gas lighter is another example. If a quartz crystal is compressed, electricity is produced. So, in the gas lighter, a piece of quartz is struck a blow by a spring-loaded hammer and the result is an electric spark to light the gas. Photoelectric cells act in the visible light spectrum to modify electric current. The bimetal strip that automatically switches off your kettle when it boils reacts to heat with mechanical movement.

Dowsing Tools

Relating these analogies to dowsing, parts of we humans exist in two systems at once. The physical body and all its surroundings with which we are familiar and this other, non-physical part in its sphere of existence. Our 'pointer on the dial' is some involuntary physical movement or sensation. When dowsing, we focus on a question (or a substance to be located) and receive some physical indication by way of response. This usually involves use of some sort of tool to magnify and make more obvious whatever the small physical response may be. Different dowsers favour different tools. One of the most versatile is a simple pendulum: a small weight on a string, as illustrated in Figure 4.3.

This is held between finger and thumb and allowed to swing. In its simplest use a question is posed that only has a *yes* or *no* answer. The pendulum will swing in one way for a yes and in some other way for a no.

Another popular tool is a pair of angle rods. These are particularly useful when walking about to locate something underground such as a water pipe.

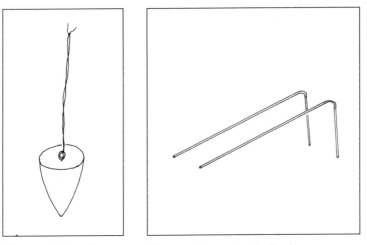

Figure 4.3 — A
Simple Pendulum

Figure 4.4 — Angle Rods

The angle rods are held one in each hand with the longer part pointing forward and parallel to the ground, shoulder width apart. The dowser walks forward while focussing attention on the object of search. The skill of visualisation, (*see* Chapter 3), comes in useful here: the clearer the mental picture of what the dowser is looking for, the more likely he is to find it and not become confused by other things detectable in the same area. On crossing the object the rods will swing both inwards, or sometimes both outwards. There are other types of tool such as the forked twig (Y-rod), or a weight on a piece of springy wire called a Bobber. All these tools serve to magnify some small involuntary muscular movement so that perception is simple.

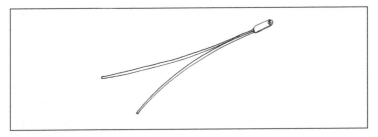

Figure 4.5 — The Forked Twig or Y-Rod

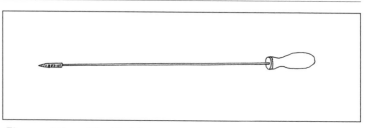

Figure 4.6 — The Bobber

The control system in the body that makes this movement is not voluntary. People observe muscles working in the lower arm and hand and say, 'You're doing it deliberately', but this is not so. The dowser is allowing an unconscious mechanism to manifest. This mechanism is most obviously seen when someone is sleepwalking: they are moving about, but not under conscious control. The mechanism runs the workings of the body over which we have little or no direct control — such as digestion — as well as the limbs and facial muscles. We can consciously make some alterations to our physical functions — e.g. breathe more deeply — but without very advanced esoteric training we cannot go far in this direction. However, it is possible to inhibit the small muscular movements that help us to dowse. We can tense up the appropriate muscles voluntarily so that they are not allowed to move, and then say it doesn't work! It can also happen at an unconscious level, due to nervousness, or to a fear that if it **does** work, a whole new way of seeing the world beyond the scientific materialistic basis will have to be contemplated. That's scary stuff for some, even if they are saying they want to learn to dowse.

Some people will tell you that a pendulum will swing in a particular way to say *yes* and another way to say *no*. In our experience, different people have different responses. One of the first things the beginner has to do is to find out what his or her particular responses are. These need to be checked at the beginning, and then regularly during a dowsing session as they can change! We also find it important to ensure that one always dowses with one's body in the same position. When using a pendulum, always use the same hand and keep it to the same side of the body. This is because the body has a polarity. It will be found that the *yes* and *no* responses will be different if the pendulum is held in one hand and used on one side of the body compared to being used crossed-over to the other side. This is important if clarity is to be maintained! We find on our courses that this is often a cause of muddle with our students. We sometimes get them to work in pairs. The dowser may have their partner sitting on their left while using the pendulum in their right hand. This is fine. But as the exercise progresses the dowser tends to turn more and more to the left toward their partner. The results of the dowsing begin to be inconsistent and confusing and we are asked for clarification. We are usually able to point out that the dowser has now got their arm crossed-over to the left side near their partner and that their responses have consequently reversed without them noticing. As soon as they return to an uncrossed posture, order is restored!

Helpful Devices

Some dowsers use other devices as well. One is a Mager Wheel. This is a small disc about three inches in diameter, which is divided into different coloured segments. A particular colour is held between finger and thumb while dowsing with whatever tool is in use. The dowsing response may be different depending on which colour segment is selected. By this means the dowser may be able to determine the quality of (say) water that he is investigating. It may be that a reaction to the water when holding the blue segment could indicate a pure drinkable supply and that black indicated impure. Another tool used by some is a Bovis Biometer. In essence this is a graduated scale and may be used in conjunction with a pendulum. While focussed on the problem in hand, the pendulum is moved along the scale until a reaction is found at some point. The graduation where the reaction is found is a numerical value related to the problem. For example, one might seek to find the strength of an earth energy line by this method. However, we do not think that the values obtained are absolute in the way that a voltmeter will give a similar result, regardless of who is using it. Values measured by a Bovis Biometer may well be useful to a dowser for comparative purposes, but may not relate to values obtained by another dowser. In any case, if one wants to get a numerical value, one could use any old ruler as a set of numbers.

We do not find these additional devices particularly useful: it is much easier to run through a counting routine in one's head, (or, if necessary, on paper), and note when the pendulum reacts. The results seem to be just as good. Similarly, we will determine quality by asking questions that have a *yes* or *no* answer directly, rather than selecting a colour on a Mager Wheel and then wondering what the significance of that colour might be. However, these devices are in essence an aid to focussing clearly on the matter in hand. Each dowser will have to find the best way for themselves and if these additional tools are found to be helpful, then by all means use them.

Clarity

So now we come to the most important aspect of all in dowsing: clarity of one's focus of attention. Another way of describing this is unambiguity in asking the question to which an answer is required. This applies whether one is using a pendulum to try and find an appropriate aromatherapy oil to use, or to walking about a site to detect some particular feature. A pendulum will give either a *yes* or a *no* response to a question. Therefore it is no good asking, 'What colour?' is something. One must ask 'Is it green?', 'Is it red?' etc. until a *yes* is obtained rather than a *no*. While site dowsing for, say, a sewer, one must keep a focus of intent on a sewer. If not one may find the water main instead, or an earth energy feature, or even just water in an underground spring. Thus, it is vital to be very clear indeed if errors are to be avoided. There is a saying about computers, 'Rubbish in, rubbish out'. This applies very much to dowsing too. If you do not ask the right question very clearly, you will not get the right answer! We treat our dowsing questioning with the same pedantic simplicity that is needed with a computer.

Concept

From the above comes the notion that if you do not have a concept of what you are seeking, then you cannot dowse for it successfully. Why not? Because if you do not have a concept you cannot frame a clear set of questions to which a yes or no response can be given.

So, to establish the pattern of earth energy at a place, one must have some sort of a framework concept in mind. Not all dowsers will agree on what this framework might be! As far as we are concerned, the end product is to be able to heal (transmute) the energies from unhelpful to helpful. Keeping our framework concept as simple as we can fulfils this aim most effectively. We do not discount that the earth energy system may, in fact, be much more complex — perhaps it is, and many dowsers do find great complexity. But while these complexities can be very interesting, they may not be relevant to being able to carry out healing work. After all, it is not necessary to know all the subtleties of the valve gear timing in the engine to be able to drive a car competently.

We have built up our framework concept from the principles taught to us by Bruce MacManaway. The principles we use are as follows: earth energy lines are straight, they have a defined width, direction of energy flow and a quality. Figure 4.7 shows a typical sketch plan of the ground floor layout of a house as an example. Two earth energy lines and a sink place are shown. We use the term sink place to denote an earth energy point rather than an earth energy line. These points can also be positive or negative and have as similar an effect on people as the lines. But they seem to be very localised, typically about one or two feet across. When dowsing on a sketch plan we always start by writing the client's name and address on the paper. We feel that this is important to help us to key into the energies of the place in relation to its inhabitants. It is conceivable that a different pattern of energy lines might be found if the people were different. For healing to be effective one needs to tune into energies at the appropriate level for the people.

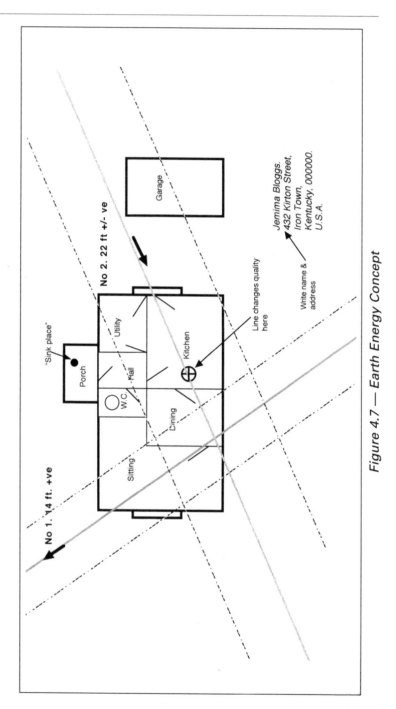

Figure 4.7 — Earth Energy Concept

We normally only draw in the centres of the energy lines, then establish the quality and the width. This is all we need for healing work. However, the figure shows the edges of the energy lines as well to indicate that, in this case, a band of effect takes in most of the house. But the effects will be most intense on the centre and edges. It will be seen that line number two is shown with a change of quality within the area of the house. This is not uncommon. So, when checking quality it is important to ask both negative and positive questions. If the response is yes to both, then we must look for the place of change within the house and establish where is the positive section and where is the negative.

When working on-site, the width can be found by dowsing while walking across the line at right angles. We get three dowsing reactions that are like crossing a road. There is an edge, the centre line and then the far edge. When doing healing work on-site, such as by driving an iron stake into the ground or placing a crystal, it is vital to be able to differentiate between the edges and the centre line. Bruce maintained that much more than a tenth of an inch out would make your work useless. The likely result of a misplaced stake would be to bend the line rather than to heal it, thus making matters worse and possibly affecting other properties. The direction of energy flow and quality we find just by asking simple questions. We follow Bruce's advice, that it is important to be out of the influence of the line when dowsing for these qualities to avoid interference leading to inaccuracies, so a map dowse before visiting the site is essential to discover where not to stand when we get there.

We use the shorthand *positive* and *negative* to describe qualities of the energy. This is not to be taken as electrical polarity. Positive lines enhance qualities such as health, happiness, harmony etc., while negative lines encourage disease, depression, disharmony and similar aspects. When checking on the quality of each earth energy line, it is advisable to check this throughout the space being considered. The quality may change for no immediately apparent reason and it may be important to establish the position of any such change to be able to effect healing work satisfactorily.

In considering the qualities of earth energies, one needs to be aware of their effect on people. Thus, when asked to dowse for the energies of a place, we usually need to know who lives there, or at least the name of the owner, and make sure that we have adequate permission for the work to be done (*see* Chapter 9). We therefore ask our dowsing questions in relation to this person as we are seeking healing to promote compatibility between the energies of place and the residents.

In addition to the earth energy features, the effect of presences and the influence of various electromagnetic radiations need to be considered. These are dealt with in other chapters.

When students are site dowsing on our courses, they will often ask, 'I get a reaction here, what is it?' Our response is 'Well, what question did you have in mind'. The usual answer is, 'Oh, I didn't have anything particular in mind!' The solution may then be to use a pendulum to ask a series of questions such as, 'Is it water, is it in a pipe, is it a supply, is it a drain, is it unpiped underground water, is it an earth energy feature, is it a gas pipe, is it an electric cable, telephone wire etc.' In our experience nearly all problems with dowsing can be traced to a lack of clarity in focussing precisely on what is required.

Map Dowsing

We do most of our work using map dowsing. This is very useful as it avoids much time and energy being used up in going to places and walking about. Map dowsing can be used to locate leaks in gas and water pipes, breaks in electric power lines, location of various underground features such as oil, minerals, archaeological remains and so on. The maps can be regular printed ones or very often a sketch plan of the area under consideration can be used. Obviously the scale needs to be appropriate for the job in hand. It will be no good trying to find the precise location to drill for water using a road atlas! Dowsers have various ways of going about map dowsing. One way is to divide the area into squares and find the appropriate square by dowsing to see if it contains the feature being sought. The square can then be subdivided again and again until a pinpoint is established. Another way is to move a pointer along one edge of the map, dowsing the while, until a reaction is obtained. This can indicate that a line drawn across the map at this point will pass through the object of the search. Do the same procedure along one of the other edges, draw a line across the map and the intersection of the two lines should be the location sought. Both these methods are useful for finding an item, e.g. a stolen car or a lost object.

When we start to investigate a request for healing a sick house, we focus on the name and address and go through a checklist (*see* Appendix 2). It covers the number of energy lines or spot features, and whether they are positive or negative. Then we check for presences and power objects (*see* chapter 6) and whether they are helpful or unhelpful to the inhabitants. It is in those areas where we can offer our healing if necessary. Then we go on to check aspects about which we would be able to offer advice and/or ongoing referral: such as adverse effects from domestic electricity, internal microwaves (by which we mean TVs and computers, occasionally ovens), external microwaves (transmission beams of some kind), water (both in pipes and underground) and airborne gases. The water problem may be interior or exterior to the house, and it may be chemical, or *informational* as discussed in Chapter 1 concerning the work of Alan Hall.

Most of our healing work is concerned with earth energies, which are usually identified as lines. Thus, a slightly different technique from the one for finding lost objects is used. We use a straight edge and lay it on the diagram. Then we ask a series of questions while rotating the straight edge until dowsing tells us it is oriented parallel to the line feature. Having established which edge of the straight edge is to be used we then ask further questions as the ruler is moved left or right, until it coincides with the line of the earth energy and then we mark the line with

a pencil. When using this technique it is important to ask for the
position of the centre line of the earth energy. Otherwise you
may find the edge instead, and some of them are many feet
wide. If the straight edge is just thrown down on the plan without conscious thought it is surprising how often it is very near
the final position. We believe that the act of putting the straight
edge down can itself be a dowsing reaction on many occasions.
After many years of this work Roy now usually 'sees' the line on
the paper and puts the straight edge down on it. On most occasions he gets it in one, but he always checks and so does Ann,
as we always work as a pair when doing this type of work. We
find it invaluable to have a second opinion always available: mistakes or misunderstandings are more readily noticed. When we
started doing this work Roy was coming more from an intellectual standpoint, Ann through intuition. For beginners it is helpful to have one of each in a team, and then grow into gnowing,
where both members of the team are using both aspects.

Differing Results

One of the difficulties conventional scientists have with dowsing
is the lack of consistency when several dowsers are involved in
the same project. Thus, they tend to dismiss the whole process
due to poor repeatability. We have found that, when dowsing for
earth energies, dowsers will often come up with different patterns for the same site. If the objective is to heal, or transmute,
the harmful energies then the dowser doing the healing should
use the pattern they found for the work. If another dowser found
a different pattern, but used that for their healing, both are likely to be effective. They may be attuned to different aspects of the
situation, or be using a different type of visualisation as a framework. This is all very confusing, but if the object of achieving
beneficial results is realised, no matter. The proof of the pudding
is in the eating!

Ann sees this from the point of view of her training and experience in psychology and psychotherapy. The differences
seem entirely right to her, but she notices that some people do

want others to agree with their own findings, as if there was something finite to be discovered when dowsing the subtle. If you are looking for drinkable water, or a lost object, it has to be finite: it's either there where you dowsed it, or it isn't, and feedback is obvious. This suits the scientific paradigm, as there is a material, factual result; even if the means to getting there is a scientific anomaly. It seems that seeing things differently where there is no direct feedback is just about inevitable, except for beginners who tend to pick up what their teacher has found. Check back to our reference on lateral thinking in the work of Edward de Bono in Chapter 3.

To complicate matters further, some attitudes to the matter in hand will affect the *truth* of findings whether thought out vertically or laterally. It is extremely difficult to set up scientific experiments that are entirely without bias; they have to start with a hypothesis on which to work anyway. The individual's background experience, be it geopathic stress, sacred space or whatever will form part of their concepts on which their dowsing is based.

The role you are playing when focussing on dowsing will also make a difference: are you trying to help someone who has black streams or negative earth energies through their house, or are you enjoying detecting some lines of energy at a sacred site? Are you doing it for healing work, or for the pleasure of detection? Travelling in our car the other day, we both remarked on something at the same time: Roy grumbled about a badly parked lorry which spoiled his sightline at a junction, Ann remarked on the beauty of a wisteria growing on a cottage wall nearby. It was his responsibility to drive safely. As a passenger she could indulge in the pleasure of admiring attractive flowers. We were both making observations from almost exactly the same position, but had seen entirely different things. This often happens in dowsing.

Sometimes when we are doing our healing-sick-houses work people send us sketch maps with lines or other dowsed features already marked on them. We find this inhibits our work, as we are not able to heal using other people's dowsed diagnosis. It seems to work when the person(s) doing the healing dowse the features on which they will base that healing themselves. This could apply to an individual dowser/healer, or to us as a couple, as we always do this work together. When working in our apprentice group, the healing can only be done if we obtain a consensus among the members, based on the diagnosis as seen by the person leading the healing.

So seeing things differently can be deemed highly subjective, but if that's the way we get results, that is how it has to be done. After all, the tools we use are only like the hands on a clock, the mechanism is within the psyche of the dowser, and these are all uniquely different, and wonderfully so. There is no way we can be boxed into identical observations or behaviours.

Chapter 5

HEALING

A definition of healing: 'Becoming more whole and sharing that wholeness with others', was offered to us by Bruce MacManaway. The words whole, heal and holy have a common history. Becoming more whole is a possible human experience, often encouraged at all levels, so it follows that we can all offer to share it if we so choose — we are all potential healers. The simplest gesture can express that sharing, such as a hand on the shoulder of someone who is distressed, or a mother rubbing her child's hurt knee. Basically, what we are offering is an energy which can flow through us because we are open to provide a channel for unconditional love.

Most people have a sense of that occurring: it's when we are focussed and allowing the flow: it seems divinely easy rather than a human struggle. It has something to do with inspiration, a word which means breathing in the spirit. An artist or a writer can focus on a subject, and the picture or words come readily to mind, but only if their channel is open and they have done enough to master the processes and techniques that will manifest their work. Healers focus their attention on the person who has asked for healing and, knowing something of the mechanisms whereby the appropriate subtle changes can affect that person, allows that universal energy to come through and activate a more whole state. It works for animals and places too.

Where does this energy come from? Everywhere! Going back to the diagrams in Chapter 3, we all have an inner core of spirituality that can connect with all-that-is. These concepts tend to go beyond words and get bogged down in cultural and religious frameworks. If we mention God, or Allah, or Jehovah, or the Universal Spirit, or Unconditional Love, or Nature, or Beings of Light, or You Name It, it is so easy for habits of thought and attitudes to diminish what is being conveyed. We have taken to calling it 'Upstairs' just to get away from those historical entanglements. Our friend, the author Hamish Miller refers to 'The Management'.

We sometimes have people telling us of their concerns that our work is not Christian. Unfortunately over the ages, various religious leaders have tried to reserve power for themselves and to dominate others under the guise of God's Word, and we do not believe that this was ever Christ's intention. Roy was born into a strictly Christian family, and went to a school where chapel attendance was frequent and compulsory. A truly significant event for Ann was her Church of England confirmation, when she was given the text, 'Stir up the gift of God which is in thee by the laying on of my hands' (2 Timothy 1:6). The Bishop's hands resting (very heavily) on her head seem to have stirred up something in her which she was later to find ways of channelling to other people. Since those early days our religious frameworks have become a great deal broader without losing, indeed while enhancing, that original spark. We all have that flame within us and, once we have recognised it, we can use it in different ways. We do not want to confine the spiritual framework within which we work to any particular doctrine, or to restrict the freedom of thought and action of others who are doing effective work. The fact that there are earth energies and associated matters that affect people, (and other life forms), helpfully or unhelpfully, is not the prerogative of any particular religious doctrine any more than electricity is. Nurturing the gift to be able to do something about the unhelpful aspects in our living conditions through spiritual healing is, in some form, within most religions. The Christian approach is the one with which we feel most comfortable. Receiving help from the divine source in the guise of any religious framework is achieved by a tightly focussed meditative process, which we would otherwise describe as intense prayer.

Following her startling experience of remote viewing (*see* Chapter 3) Ann explored gradually, within the limitations of caring for our family, further and further into our new understandings outside the 'normal' scientific and religious paradigms of the time. She talked with members of the Theosophical Society, which had a major lodge in Camberley, and through them met up with wonderful people at the College of Psychic Studies in London (*see* Appendix 1, Resources): Paul Beard, Bill Blewett, Cynthia Lady Sandys and many others, who felt that she had been given this awareness of another dimension in order to become a healer. Some literature was available — only a minute amount compared with today — and she read avidly. She worked with several healers, including Harry Edwards for a while. Harry Edwards had done more to encourage the recognition of spiritual healing than any others in those early days. The Witchcraft Act was repealed only in 1952 and, although it hadn't been exercised for many years before then, there was still a notion of illegality and being out of tune with cultural norms if healing was administered other than within medical parameters, or as part of church ritual. The National Federation of Spiritual Healers (*see* Appendix 1, Resources) came into being to make this kind of work more acceptable and respectable, and has gone from strength to strength. Ann was one of the first to be named on their Healer Register.

Dowsing has had a bad press with the Church because it was seen as divining. Being outside our normal three-dimensional universe, and therefore in need of special protective measures (*see* Chapter 9), it was not to be undertaken by just anybody. Dowsing for water was excepted for practical reasons. This attitude is now changing as we have found in personal discussions with clergy, and by the fact that a number of ministers have attended our courses. Dowsing is a natural ability possessed by virtually everybody and is no more than a methodical way of tapping into your own intuition. Our intuitive awareness is a way of accessing the universal store of knowledge since we are all connected into that Oneness.

Healers give focussed attention to the needs of someone or something specific, then connect with Upstairs in whatever way they see It, and ask that whatever is necessary and appropriate be done. It's really that simple! What we humans find so difficult is the focussing and the connecting, and that is what takes training and practice. We are so conditioned to rely on our own wits and expertise and physical dexterity, that just setting the scene and leaving it to Upstairs can feel impossible. Ann recollects a lesson about that: she says,

'I have an unstable situation in my lower back, so it "goes out", occasionally — very painful and disabling. When it happened one day just as I was about to go out and fetch my young children from school, I was in a real fix. I lay on the floor and shouted, "Help", to Upstairs, as I could think of no way I could help myself or retrieve my children safely. There was nothing I, as a human being, could do. Within a minute or two I was moving my back, and very shortly I was driving, pain free, to the school. I only had to admit my complete helplessness and ask.'

One of the basic premises of healing is to get out of the way! It is so easy to **want** something to happen, to think we know what should happen, but that actually inhibits the process of healing. Many healers ask some source to which they feel attuned, to do the healing through and for them in order to avoid this interference. They use guides or talismans, (*see* Chapter 9), which effectively takes the human personality out of the act. It's like opening a doorway, and allowing what needs to happen, what is right in a given circumstance, to come into manifestation with less difficulty.

In very mundane terms, healing is a bit like using jump leads to help start a car whose battery has run down. Connections are made which allow the energy needed to pass from one vehicle to the other. The *healer* car has its engine running and is therefore connected to a power source with its battery being charged, so that it is not depleted itself. In the context of our opening definition, it is as whole as it can be, and is then sharing its wholeness with the other car. It is using energy that it can pass through to another, not running down its own battery. This is a very important consideration in this kind of healing work. Sharing his or her wholeness does not deplete the healer; indeed many actually feel that they gain something in the process. Imagine the healer being like a pipe curved at right angles, when he or she connects to Upstairs and then to the subject in front of them, the pipe opens to the energy from above which pours through. Some of it rubs off on the pipe on the way!

Healer training now involves an element of studying anatomy and physiology. It is not that healers are required to diagnose — indeed it is unwise to do so — but a certain basic knowledge permits an understanding of the patients' state of health as they describe their symptoms and difficulties. Ann had a head start in this respect as her father was a GP in rural Herefordshire, with the surgery and dispensary in her home. So she was absorbed a great deal with health and the way people deal with any lack of it. There can also be an advantage if the healer has known illness, and possibly faced his or her own mortality, provided the implications of this experience have been worked through so the healer's own reactions are not imposed on other people. Ann's principle relevance to this was her own very serious illness in her late teens, necessitating two years of in-patient treatment and carrying a very poor prognosis at the time of diagnosis. By knowing what it feels like to be lacking in health and likely to die, the healer can do a better job.

Connecting to Wholeness

We start from the premise that there is potentially a perfect wholeness, to which we can all aspire, yet being unlikely to reach it while in a physical body. The experience that led Ann to hold this hypothesis happened in a very unpromising hospital situation. She was sitting with a dying friend. The doctors had withdrawn all support mechanisms, awaiting the end, and 'Les' was clearly very poorly indeed. Seeking to ease his passage to the next world, Ann asked him if he had recently seen Henry, a special person of 'Les's' acquaintance who was not in our world.

'Les's' eyes lit up, he sat up and asked for a drink. When he had enjoyed that, he lay back on the bed and, to Ann's perception, changed into a *perfect* version of himself, young and in blooming health. He died shortly thereafter. Ann took this vision to be 'Les's' ideal self, his archetype for this life, the total potential of his wholeness. One way of looking at our state on earth is to see that perfection projected into the physical, in a similar way to an architect's design becoming a building. He or she draws it in an ideal state, then a few snags occur in the building, so it turns out not exactly as originally drawn. After years of wear and tear the building deteriorates, various maintenance and repair jobs are done, until at some stage it becomes too damaged to be viable any more. If that is the case, then the healer is making connection with the architect's design, strengthening its ability to reform the human being nearer to its perfect state. Linking with Upstairs in this way improves wholeness.

This linking could be seen in terms of frequencies and harmonics. There are resonances between levels of awareness, rather like octaves on the piano, (of which there are seven!), which can provide us with a stairway between the most mundane and the most spiritual levels. By accessing that hierarchy of frequencies the healer facilitates the means whereby wholeness can be more readily approached. Many skilled and gifted healers are using actual sound, with musical instruments or with their own voices, to establish connection. Finding your own specific frequency has wonderful healing potential.

Making these healing connections, sharing our wholeness, is something everyone can do if they wish. Some people are naturals at it — to use a musical analogy, they are prodigies like Mozart. Others need to work much harder at it — they are more like those who are deemed tone deaf and told to stand at the back and mouth the words in the school choir. Actually, they just need to release that blockage and let the energy flow through their voices. Letting it flow is the clue, whether we are talking about sound or healing coming through.

People refer to faith healing as if you have to believe in something, or have a specific religious faith, to make it work for you. The only faith the recipient of this healing energy needs to have is that it is likely to help them; i.e. they are open to receiving it. If they have taken the trouble to visit a healer, or have asked for some help at a distance, whether for themselves or for their place, then the channel (the pipe) is likely to be open enough for the healing energy to get through. Sometimes ingrained inhibitions make this difficult, but with patience and discussion this is usually overcome. The safeguard is that if someone doesn't want to receive healing, whatever they may be saying on the surface to please others or to meet peer pressure, it will not get through to them, so there is no risk of intrusion.

Chakras

If we look at the aura, the etheric, the energy body, or whatever you like to call it; we can gain some ideas about how Upstairs reaches the human being living on earth in order to effect healing. The system of vortices or centres of energy, called *chakras*, within the aura but co-existent with the physical body, comes from Eastern cultures and is now more widely known in the West. Correlations are made between the chakras and the glands of the hormonal system, as links between the subtle and the material. There are now many books about this system, some with beautiful pictures of the chakras as seen by clairvoyants, and depicted by artists (especially in the form of halos for very spiritual beings). Our diagram (Figure 5.1) is hugely simplistic, and we will just make a few comments which may be helpful in understanding healing rather than treat the subject in depth (*see* Bibliography and References, Section 9).

We suggest that each human being lives in a column of subtle energy, from under our feet to well above our heads. The crown chakra at the top of our heads and the base chakra, (sited on the perineum, the area below the end of the spine on which we sit), remain open to connect us between heaven and earth. The five in between, (how often we come up with sevens!), can to a certain extent, and with practice, be controlled by the person living in them. The five chakras in between can also be

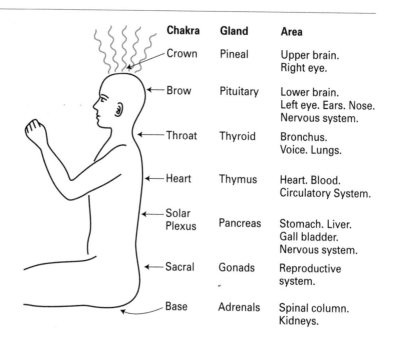

Chakra	Gland	Area
Crown	Pineal	Upper brain. Right eye.
Brow	Pituitary	Lower brain. Left eye. Ears. Nose. Nervous system.
Throat	Thyroid	Bronchus. Voice. Lungs.
Heart	Thymus	Heart. Blood. Circulatory System.
Solar Plexus	Pancreas	Stomach. Liver. Gall bladder. Nervous system.
Sacral	Gonads	Reproductive system.
Base	Adrenals	Spinal column. Kidneys.

Figure 5.1 — Correlation between Chakras and Glands

affected by outside influences. Wholeness is about these vortices or centres being energised in an optimal fashion and in balance with each other — more open or more closed to suit the prevailing environmental situation. There is constant change. As the vicissitudes of earthly life impinge on this delicate balance, wholeness may be compromised. For some this is a burdensome situation affecting balance from an early age, for others the habits of being out of balance develop more slowly. By sharing their wholeness, healers can reconnect people with their perfect, whole aspect, i.e. their architect's drawing, and the situation takes a step toward improvement.

Traditionally healers have used their hands to channel this gift from Upstairs. Our everyday gestures of comfort are most often using hands, and the Christian tradition uses the laying on of hands. There are secondary centres in the palms of the hands, connected to the heart chakra. So, this is the area of our column of subtle energy that we can most readily open to extend unconditional love to another being. The healer may also, or instead, be speaking or making sound, and this is channelling via the throat chakra. We do this when speaking kindly to someone, or singing to a fractious baby. The brow chakra, manifesting through the eyes, is another channel for healing, and can be used when the other two would not be appropriate; for example, in an emergency or hospital situation when it is important not to get in the way of healers working at a more physical level. Again, in more everyday situations, a glance of sympathy or a focussed visualisation can be very helpful. The only difference between these everyday gestures and an act of healing is one of scale, intensity and focussed intent. Healers have learned and practised to cultivate themselves as wide and pure a *pipe* for the channelling as they can manage for the moment, and have some skill in opening and shutting the necessary taps to facilitate the flow of energy from Upstairs and send it in the appropriate direction.

Directing the Healing

Where it is going is just as important as where it comes from. It might be generally beneficial to spread this wonderful energy in all directions, and people with very strong connections with Upstairs who can do this are hugely appreciated — e.g. the Pope with his blessing, 'Urbi et omni'. But for most of us we need to focus where we are sending it so that it doesn't become too diluted to be effective, more like a laser beam than a general diffusion of light. This is why healers are most effective when they link strongly with the person or place they are seeking to help. Probably this is simplest when they are physically present and in touch. Healers sometimes place their hands on a person's clothed skin, especially if there is physical pain, but more often work an inch or two away from the body, where they can sense the aura. It is perfectly possible to send healing by holding a person's hand, and channelling via the chakra centres in the palms.

However, being in touch can happen at a distance, any distance, and much healing is given in this way. Some people would call it prayer. A great deal of research has been undertaken into the effectiveness of healing prayer (*see* Bibliography and References 6.2). Some kind of linking object, or *witness* such as a photograph or a letter, in addition to the person's name, is helpful to strengthen the focus for the healer.

For our work in healing sick houses we need the person's name and address, and a sketch map of their home, as described in Chapter 4 and, of course, their permission. It is useful to have a letter about why they thought their place needed healing, or some notes of a phone conversation when they told their story. Some people send area maps and photos that certainly help to put us in the picture, but these are not essential. We do need to be in touch with both the place and the people living there, because the healing is about making the place more compatible with the people, not about a finite kind of positive environment which would suit everyone. We feel this is a very important aspect of our work: we notice that some dowsers are engineering subtle environments into a state which they believe to be universally right, but we think different people need different subtle environments in which they can flourish and become more whole. It's rather like different people needing different kinds of dwelling places at a physical level: one family would be best suited in a detached house in the country, another would feel more whole in an urban flat. So, we all need to live and work in an atmosphere which nourishes us at a subtler level.

Some of our clients take a while to get used to the new subtle environment when we have healed their place, the change feels strange, and they only start to feel the benefit when they have settled into the new state of their home. For some it works like a homoeopathic remedy: they feel briefly worse before getting better. For others the improvement is slow and only noticed with hindsight. If they have been ill and depleted by negative earth energies for a long time, it takes a while for their batteries to recharge, and we often suggest they find someone to give them spiritual healing personally as well, and/or we offer distant healing ourselves.

We think that the qualities of the place where healing is carried out is important for good results. We usually do all our work in Ann's study/consulting room, which has a very good atmosphere. One of the reasons that we came to live in this house is because of the very powerful and beneficial earth energy lines running through the house and garden. We will write more about this in Chapter 8.

It can be difficult to grasp the fact that things are changing all the time. There is no finite state of health, of people or places, which will endure. Listen to a piece of music you know well with a critical ear: you will notice a wrong note or some mistiming, which is there and gone again within that second of time. It has happened, and cannot be gone over again, at least only by replaying the phrase later. The vibration has emerged and been manifest in an imperfect form. Here the design of the composer, rather than the architect, has been to some extent distorted, but the music continues and the whole piece has its own validity even if it doesn't come out exactly as planned. This is a useful analogy for life in all its forms. Nothing is static. A valid healing act causes a step function in the process, which then triggers other reactions and events.

Healing of Places

When we first started healing sick houses under the instruction of Bruce, the process was simple and down to earth. He only taught people who were already healers, and used to finding their own inner strength, reaching to Upstairs and channelling the energy required. He instructed us in dowsing so that we could establish a focus for healing the selected place. First, we dowsed remotely for lines on a map supplied by the client, as described in Chapter 4; then we travelled to the place and found out exactly where the lines were on the ground. On his courses this exercise took on a happy atmosphere of an expedition or field trip, with everyone giving their view, so that we eventually came to a consensus about what to do in the way of healing. Then Bruce opened the boot of his large car, revealing lengths of heavy angle iron and a sledgehammer. We dowsed for the length of metal to be used on each negative line, and then banged it into the ground in **exactly** the right place, defined by dowsing. The aspect of the healing which needed good focus and intent was fulfilled by the effort required by the person wielding the sledgehammer, and if possible the owner of the property was asked to at least start this action, even if someone stronger had to finish it off. The whole exercise had a communal interactive feel about it, with the owners as well as the healer(s) involved.

By contrast, the remote work we now do (for the development of this, *see* Chapter 2) is usually just us two, although we can involve our regular healing or teaching groups if necessary. Sometimes members bring cases in need of additional attention from their own practice. These are closed groups — i.e. of committed members who come to nearly every meeting, not casual people who just drop in when they feel like it, and this is important for maintaining cohesion in the energies of those present for effective healing work. Our highly focussed meditative process now constitutes the intent needed, and takes the place of the angle iron and sledgehammer technique: easier physically, but a lot harder at mental and intuitive levels!

For some years, in both these modes, it took some hours for the energies to clear through. It was as if we had done something to clear a blockage in a river, and the flow rearranged itself as the impetus travelled downstream. This could be uncomfortable for the inhabitants of the place, and we warned them of the possibility of minor disturbances like headaches, tummy upsets, fractious children. Then in 1996, Roy had the opportunity to visit Mother Meera, a special avatar person born in India and now living in Germany. He sought her blessing on behalf of both of us, and Ann felt this back home in Somerset. Roy did not notice much at the time, but the next healing job we did occurred instantaneously, with no time to clear through, so something had happened to render the healing channel more effective. Almost all house healings have needed no time to clear since this experience, and we are awe-fully grateful for this improvement for the sake of our clients.

We know a number of healers who call on living gurus such as Mother Meera or Sai Baba to help them with their work. Others have Guides or Helpers, sometimes named or recognised. We are pragmatic: we use whatever works! Beings of Light, the Christ Spirit or the Divine Source, seem right for us; or just *Upstairs*.

Chapter 6

PRESENCES

What do we mean by presences? They can take many forms. It is not uncommon for people to report that they sense somebody is looking at them, except that there is nobody to be seen. A typical request from a client might be, 'My little girl says there is a man in her bedroom, but there is no-one there. Can you get rid of him?' We hear about more physical manifestations such as odd knockings or sometimes smells. Poltergeist activity, reported as 'things moving about' to a greater or lesser extent, is also experienced on occasion. We find that these effects can have several different causes. The most common cause is by the activities of discarnate beings, by which we mean the souls, or non-physical enduring aspects of people who are now dead or who have passed on. Sometimes these are friends or loved ones who are merely interested in what is going on in the physical world and are not a problem.

The reason that we came to pay attention to these presences is that they can affect our own energy levels in a very similar way to that of earth energies. If a presence is trying to manifest in some way then it can tap into a human energy system to feed itself. We found out about presences in relation to earth energies very early on. We had been asked to deal with 'things that go bump in the night' on several occasions. We usually found harmful earth energies and would transmute them to be beneficial. This usually caused the manifestations to cease.

In one case this action did not produce the desired effect. The lady of the house had called us in to try to cure knocking noises that were heard from time to time, and some alarming movement of objects. She had already enlisted the help of another well-known dowser, but his treatment with an object placed in the house did not stop these strange phenomena. Our own findings were that the earth energies had reverted to being unhelpful and dealt with them in our usual way. The knocking noises continued. We checked up on the situation several times and found all the earth energies to be beneficial, but still the noises and movements continued. Of course, we had looked for all the more usual causes of noises such as the water in the heating system etc. Eventually we realised that the cause was something with an energy of its own, so we should be looking for an entity or presence and find out why it was making the disturbance. Why was it attracting attention? What did it want? It emerged that the lady had had two late miscarriages and then a baby who had lived only a few days. When we did further questioning by dowsing it seemed the incoming soul was disorientated by its situation. Having decided to incarnate, but now unable to have a functioning body, it then could not return to source and so had become trapped. We were able, with the help of our healing group, to encourage it reconnect with source and there was no further trouble.

More typically the presence is someone who has lived many years but is confused by no longer having a physical body. They can apparently perceive us but are unable to communicate directly or be noticed, except by people who have the appropriate kind of sixth sense. Some are still trying to work out things that were not resolved while they were alive. If this includes thoughts of revenge for some supposed wrongdoing, this can lead to more unpleasant behaviour. If people understand about life after death and know that their time is coming, then are able to prepare accordingly, all is usually well. On the other hand, for one who only considers the material existence and comes to a sudden end in an accident, then this person may feel quite lost. With no concept of an afterlife then there will not apparently be one. But the consciousness is still in existence, albeit in an unpleasant limbo state. Ann learned about this originally from some wise members of the Theosophical Society, and later from Bruce MacManaway, whose mother was very active in this field.

A great deal of visualisation and healing work had been done during the First World War, and subsequently, to assist young men killed in battle who were wandering around in another state of existence, confused and miserable. The visualisation often used by the Theosophical Society members was of a barracks where they could learn more about their situation, and move on in the hierarchy of existences. They called this kind of intervention rescue work. It seems that souls who are stuck need someone in incarnation to introduce them to Beings of Light or some other appropriate entity or discarnate soul for guidance in moving on. Many presences in houses are simply asking for a helpful introduction, so they are drawn to people sensitive to such levels of existence, and their manifestation is often made easier in an environment where there are negative earth energies. There are many books now available that describe these sort of events (*see* Bibliography and References, Section 2).

Terry and Natalia O'Sullivan (*see* Bibliography and References 2.5) have made extensive researches into the spirit world and its interactions with our own. In the course of these investigations they have travelled widely and sought out the views and beliefs of people from many different cultures. Within many eastern and indigenous peoples, an acknowledgement and understanding of the spirit world is commonplace. In their travels, the O'Sullivans have found that there seem to be more lost souls giving problems in communities with a monotheistic religion than in those that believe in reincarnation. These are primarily Christianity, Islam and Judaism, which all stem from a common root. These religions do not now subscribe to reincarnation, (it was outlawed by the Christian Church in the fourth century by the Nicean Council), and are inclined to see lost souls as demons. Their teachings on states of existence after physical death are not particularly helpful as it is suggested that the destination is either eternal bliss in heaven or eternal damnation in hell. It is therefore not surprising that many fear death and are not prepared for the situation that they find themselves in after physical death of the body.

The Rev

Even those who one would expect to know where they were going after passing over cannot always resist taking an interest in what goes on in the world after their death. We have an example here at our home: our architect-designed bungalow was built to the order of a retired minister in the early 1930s. It obviously meant a lot to him. We were told by one of his relatives living nearby that he wished to be able to absorb the view across the Somerset Levels to Glastonbury Tor for the rest of his days — he even had the sitting-room built on the north side of the house to facilitate this. We made his acquaintance due to poltergeist activity: the cistern in the toilet was prone to misbehave not long after we moved in. Roy fixed the plumbing, but it didn't stay fixed as his repairs usually do. One day a young friend with a well-developed sixth sense visited, and we asked him to have a good sit there, and tell us if he could detect anything.

He emerged looking puzzled and saying it was all about a bird table! We remembered that there had been an ancient and wobbly stone bird table in the middle of the lawn, and that Roy had knocked it over with the mower several times and eventually removed it because it was inconvenient. We checked with an aerial photograph that had been given to us by the people who sold us the house and who had done an enormous amount of work on the garden. This picture had been taken when they took over from the executors to the minister's widow to show the garden before they started on it. There was the bird table, so it was obviously connected with The Rev, as we affectionately call him now. It was just a question of acknowledging that he had put a lot of thought and effort into having this place built, helping him to accept the alterations we were making; and above all, justifying our healing activities here, which he obviously thought should only happen in church. The toilet then behaved itself, and we are quite happy to have The Rev visit if

he feels like it. Further investigations revealed that the bathroom
had originally been his study, and that the toilet was placed in
the position of his desk, where the best view of Glastonbury Tor
was available. So not all *presences* intend to make trouble, they
just need to be acknowledged and to work something through.

Effects of Presences

We had an interesting example of effects on the animal kingdom
a few years ago. A farmer had asked us to look into and correct
the earth energies at her property. This we did, but found that a
large number of discarnates were also part of the problem. Our
dowsing questioning revealed that these were men who had
been killed in a battle that had take place in those parts a long
time ago: they were troubled because they had been left to die
on the ground, with no proper burial. We were able to help them
to move to their rightful sphere of existence by visualising that
proper burial, including reading the service from the old Book
of Common Prayer. When we contacted the farmer to tell her
that we had done the work, she said that she knew that we had.
On asking why, she said that her sheep would never willingly
go into one corner of one of her fields. You will have seen sheep
in a field and they are usually scattered all over fairly evenly
(unless being herded). The farmer reported that they would now
scatter themselves all over this field and no longer avoided the
corner as before.

We have found a number of effects that seem to be attribut-
able to discarnates or *lost souls*. There are, of course, often beneficial aspects such as the inspiration received by writers and
artists, which may come from these sources. Of more concern to
our work as healers are the adverse effects. These can range
from a feeling of being drained and a lack of energy, through to
quite violent behaviour. In severe cases of the latter it would
seem that the discarnate can take over control of the physical
body of a person for a time. It is not uncommon to read in the
newspapers of violent deeds being done and after the event the
perpetrator will say something like, 'I don't know what came

over me. It wasn't me.' There are psychiatrists who are now considering that some mental illnesses such as schizophrenia may be due to the effects of discarnate entities rather than some upset of the brain chemistry.

'James' came to Ann as a counselling client. He had been convicted of arson and had served some time in prison as a result. He drove about on a small motorbike and he was concerned that sometimes he felt a great urge to move to the opposite side of the road just as traffic was approaching. As soon as the potentially conflicting traffic had passed, this urge to become an accident left him. He could not account for these urges and said, 'It's not me'. He could only avoid causing an accident by considerable effort of will to overcome the urge. Not unnaturally, he was worried lest his will power might not be sufficient on one occasion. It emerged that he was one of twins but his brother had died at a young age. After some counselling, it was found by dowsing that the spirit of his dead twin was still around and trying to attract attention so as to be able to continue the broken relationship with his brother. We arranged for 'James' to meet with our healing group and together we were able to help the deceased twin's spirit to return to its rightful sphere and to stop interfering with his brother's continuing life. It was also concluded that the arson attacks resulted from the same connection. We maintained contact with 'James' for some time afterwards and he was able to pursue a normal life without any further problems of this nature.

We have found instances where the earth energies have been adversely affected by discarnates. It seems that it is easier for them to relate to the physical world at places with negative earth energies; the subtle atmospheric pull is then toward gravity and physical manifestation rather than *levity*, in the direction of spirit. So it seems that they strive to increase the negative effect in order to stay present. These findings emphasise the need to heal the presences inhabiting a place as well as the place itself; if this is not done, the house can soon become sick again, with resulting damage to any sensitive person living there.

We have also occasionally come across instances where discarnates have used the electrical system. In one case of a cottage in Wales we were asked to heal, the lady mentioned unaccountably high electricity consumption. Not only were the earth energies negative, but there was a discarnate involved as well. It turned out that her husband had died suddenly and in rather dramatic circumstances and it was not long after that when the electricity bills started to increase alarmingly, without any extra use of power by the family. Our conclusion was that the husband was trying to manifest his continuing presence as he wanted to provide his widow with a vital piece of practical information; he had been able to use the electrical energy from the supply in some way in his endeavour to manifest sufficiently clearly. After we had healed the earth energies, and dowsed for the information the discarnate husband was offering, we helped him to his appropriate sphere of existence, and the electricity consumption returned to normal.

Power Objects

'Jenny' suffered from a disabling degenerative disease. She was trying everything to become healed. We were contacted because of her concern that the energies of her rather grand house might not be helpful. Indeed there were problems and we made appropriate corrections. However, the energies returned to a negative state after a short time, so we thought that there was more to this case than usual. By dowsing, we found that there was what we now call a power object in the house that was affecting the earth energies adversely. Eventually we found that this object was a fine carved wooden lion's head that graced the newel post of their impressive staircase. This had been brought back from Africa as a curio some years ago and mounted on the newel post where it looked just fine. It is suspected that it had been 'fixed up' by a witch doctor for some purpose or other. As soon as we had identified this as the problem object, to our surprise 'Jenny's' husband produced a large saw and immediately cut the top off the post. They were advised to ritually burn the lion's head in the garden, which they did soon after.

We were always reminded of this case when visiting Jenny as, on entering the hall by the front door, one was immediately confronted by the splendid staircase with the post at the bottom looking rather out of place due to its crooked sawn-off top! There was no more trouble with the earth energies going negative subsequently. Sadly, 'Jenny's' disease had progressed too far to be reversible, but she was much happier and lived a few more years of fruitful life. Our work aroused her interest in spiritual healing, and led to her being able to channel healing herself although progressively disabled.

One of the really rewarding parts of this work is its catalytic effect: it opens more and more doors into other dimensions of human consciousness, not only for us, but for a number of our clients too. One man wrote to us instantly when he read about our work in a Sunday newspaper, asking us to check and heal his brother's house. The brother had just had a brain tumour diagnosed. It was fast growing and resulted in his death, but his healed environment meant, according to our correspondent, that he had a comfortable ending to his life, astonishing the doctors with his lack of degeneration until very near the end. We had advised personal spiritual healing which helped enormously, and after his death, the living brother took training to become a healer and is doing wonderful service.

Another example of a power object was a ceremonial sword that had pride of place on a wall in someone's hall. Our dowsing questioning found that it had belonged to a high-ranking official who had ordered the execution of a number of pirates caught in the South China Sea. The sword had not actually cut off their heads, but was representative of that authority. Finding a rightful place of existence for the brigands was not easy, and we advised the owners of the sword to put it out of the house, at least for a while. Unfortunately they gave it to their gardener, who then became ill. We did not hear the end of this story because we were not given the opportunity to cleanse the sword. We have since heard of a way of removing the energies of such charged objects from a house that we may try in the future. Someone was once advised to leave an offending object outside the entrance to their home so that it could be picked up by whoever was supposed to have it next. The karmic implications of this solution need thinking about!

We advised a lady who had a German stein, a beer mug with a lid, which was exuding unfortunate vibrations in her sitting room, to remove it from her house. She decided to take it to the local antique shop. The owner was not available so she left it for valuation. There was much embarrassment when she called again at the shop: the stein was nowhere to be found, so it had done its own disposal.

Objects can, of course, be imbued with positive energy. Obvious examples are religious objects that have been blessed by a priest.

Other Entities

There are a number of different non-physical entities other than discarnate people. Elementals, or nature spirits, can sometimes cause problems. We have only had limited experience of these in our work, but they are mentioned here as the possibility of their involvement should not be ignored. Of course, many of them are very helpful, particularly in assisting plants and trees to flourish. No doubt those gardeners who talk to their plants are addressing these helpers of Nature, and if they call them divas, they are not referring to operatic sopranos! Sometimes these spirits are displaced, perhaps by the felling of a tree, or the destruction of some area of landscape or special plant. They have been known to intrude on people or spaces because they have nowhere to live any more. The solution is to find them a suitable habitat.

We have also found that some very old houses have been given a *guardian* when they were built. An animal, usually a dog, was ritually buried in the hearth or on the threshold, and charged with caring for the place. In later years, when renovations and alterations have been made, the bones have been disturbed and the guardian made homeless, prowling around trying to get back into its rightful domain and resentful of those who caused the disturbance. In this case we advise the inhabitants to select an article which can be designated as the guardian's own space, like a kennel, and place that with intent in the hearth or on the threshold as appropriate. In doing so they should acknowledge the presence and help of the guardian. We have had some amazingly positive feedback about the effects of this small but significant act of rehabilitation.

Naturally, human beings can also affect the ambience of a place, and in turn the polarity of the earth energies. Sometimes we find a line changing from positive to negative within a house. We have to be very tactful about this, but it frequently transpires that someone has had a very significant experience at that spot such as hearing very bad news, or having a flaming row, or even a sudden death. Because they were on the centre of an earth energy line at the time, the polarity was switched.

There are many different factors in healing sick houses, and we are very likely to find more as our experience continues to expand. We think that it is probable that some of the more materially based gadgets sold to combat geopathic stress do not encompass the problem of presences or entities. This may be why we hear from a number of clients that they have tried such remedies and found that their effects did not last.

Great care is needed when addressing this area of work, which is so obviously in another dimension of awareness. It really is better not to touch it unless you know how to conduct yourself safely. We will deal with personal protection in Chapter 9.

Chapter 7

PERSONAL STORIES

We always learn a great deal from reactions reported by our clients. Some, such as the ones we present in this chapter, are very generous in giving time and attention to letting us know how they feel. Others only mention it some time later, perhaps when they move house and want us to check their new place. 'Your work on Blackberry Cottage five years ago made such a difference, we'd like you to....' Nice if they'd told us then, really! Sometimes we get someone on the phone concerned that their symptoms are worse immediately after the healing. We compare this to the effect of homoeopathic treatment. When the remedy is just right, all the symptoms exaggerate before departing. Obviously we check that the energies have stayed positive and invite the person to call again if things have not improved in a week or so. Some people find it difficult to acclimatise themselves to the change for the better in their subtle environment, just as one might find it difficult to change from damp cold Britain in wintertime to hot dry India, or adjust to a clock change when travelling round the world. We suggest they are suffering from something akin to jet lag! But very often we hear nothing: as most therapists will tell you, people get better and go away and forget about it, only coming back if they are not satisfied.

The following stories come from people whose houses we have healed — they speak for themselves.

From Margaret in Essex

'Less than a year after moving to our home I was aware of feeling more tired than usual. As the years passed my energy seemed to be constantly low, which made life restricting. A hormonal imbalance and food sensitivity added to the problems.

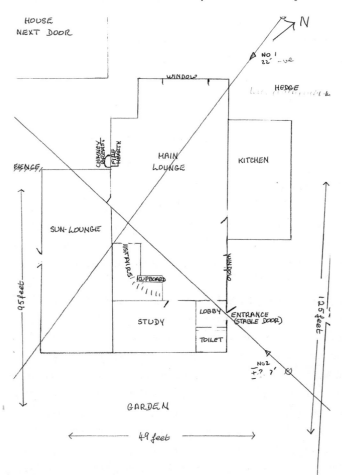

Figure 7.1 — Energy Lines at Margaret's House in Essex

Then in 1997 a friend discovered, through dowsing, that there was an underground stream directly beneath where we sleep — not good for health, I understood. However, it was another two years, and more fatigue-related problems later, that another friend put me in touch with the Procters.

'They found two negative energy lines here, and within a couple of weeks of the *House Healing* being carried out I was aware of feeling more positive and motivated than I had in a long time. Then came an increase in energy, making everyday tasks easier. I can walk up and down the stairs now without my legs feeling like lead, and I'm not so food sensitive. I am both surprised and very impressed with the results, and would highly recommend the valuable work that the Procters are doing.'

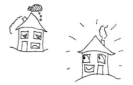

From Tessa in Hertfordshire

'In 1997 I was diagnosed with having Non-Hodgkin's Lymphoma. I soon realised that I could not have complete faith in my doctors' ability to help me recover fully, simply because they discounted the issues that I felt had led to my illness. I knew intuitively that a combination of issues had contributed to the breakdown of my immune system, and I was sure that if I could address them then I would have a better chance of recovery. So I began my journey of self-discovery. I looked at body and mind issues, in that order, not realising then that they are interconnected. I knew when I read about negative earth energies in *Caduceus* magazine that this was relevant to my situation because I had been unsettled at home for a long time. We built our house in the early 1980s on the very exposed site of a new barn very near to an electricity substation. I invited a local dowser to look at our house and he, to my amazement, detected that I was sleeping over a combination of geopathic stress lines.

However, moving bedrooms did not ease my mind or my physical demise and eventually I rang Ann and Roy for help.

'I duly sent them a very simple plan of the house. My husband spoke to Ann first because I was out at the time. He told me later that he was led, phone in hand, to my jumble cupboard over the kitchen. I was impressed at the accuracy of their guidance as they seemed to be looking for something flat like a picture on the wall. A week later Ann spoke to me and led me, again phone in hand, back to the same cupboard. I knew the contents so it didn't take long to find what we were looking for. When we located it I immediately burst into tears as it was such an emotional release. It was the Balinese shadow puppet I had bought for my husband's birthday five years previously. A

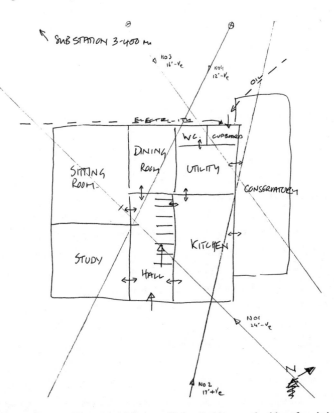

Figure 7.2 — Energy Lines at Tessa's House in Hertfordshire

couple of years later, just before my diagnosis and during a tense time between us, he had asked me to take it down from the wall as he found it rather spooky. Not wanting to dispose of it I stuffed it into a flat paper bag and put it in the cupboard. It was an amazing experience for me because it was the sign that I needed to restore my faith in God and his powers of healing. Ann was concerned because I was so emotional and she suggested I remove it from the house as soon as possible. I had a log fire burning in the hearth so I ceremoniously burnt it. I went down on my knees for I had this compulsion to pray for forgiveness for bringing it into our lives. The outcome of this incredible experience is that I now have absolute faith in prayer and divine energy that exists in us in our landscape. It is very relevant to my work as a landscape architect with healing landscapes. But most of all I am reassured in the knowledge that Ann and Roy continue to send me healing.'

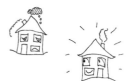

From Elena in Luxembourg

'It is difficult to put into precise words what Ann and Roy Procter have done for my home at intervals over the past few years. Difficult because I do not rightly understand it myself, and difficult because the benefits I have reaped are obviously open to accusations of subjectivity and wishful thinking.

'Neither Ann nor Roy has ever seen my home nor have we met. I contacted them through a mutual acquaintance at a time when my home was the scene of sudden domestic pain and destruction. They could not (nor pretended to) prevent the destruction but did work on the house, finding and healing acute, negative earth energy lines and interferences. From a place of conflict it became a place of strength for me.

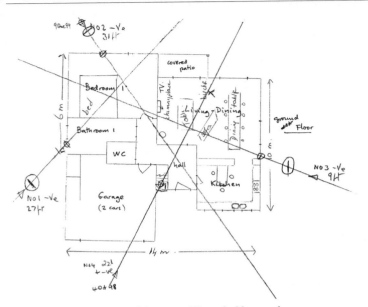

Figure 7.3 — Energy Lines at Elena's House in Luxembourg

'There have been times when this right balance has appeared disrupted. Ann and Roy have redressed this balance, offering gentle explanations as to why this fine line of health had slipped. As already said, I do not know exactly what they did, but I do know their explanations have always fitted with the facts being lived here at the time, and that I am grateful for their help.'

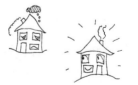

From Gwen in North Wales

'We read about you in a Sunday supplement. At point in our lives we were desperate to know why, despite being generally optimistic and positive, we just seemed to hit one crisis after another. My late sister was a healer and spent much of her time

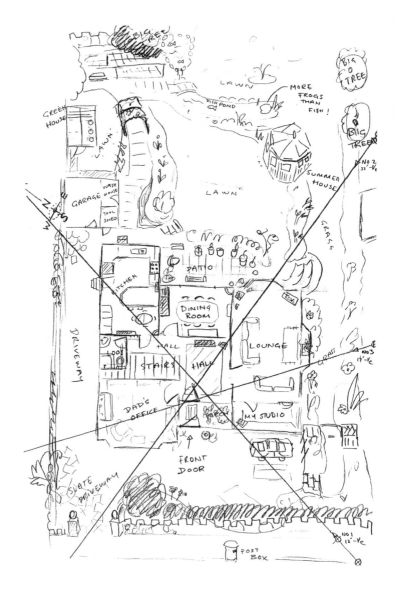

Figure 7.4 — Energy Lines at Gwen's House in North Wales

involved in healing. I am more earthy but have always believed in the power of good and that there is much more to life than we experience here.

'We needed to reach out for help and feel that someone was there — you did that and we are all very grateful. My daughter (the one who illustrates children's books and made the map for you) and I felt a *lightening* in the atmosphere which helped enormously. Some time later we felt things had deteriorated and wrote to you again. You confirmed that a line had become negative and healed us again.'

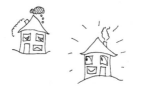

From Diana in Surrey
A tale with a happy ending...

'I had been a patient of Dr N. for some time, suffering a variety of ailments and allergies, largely due to chronic stress and all exacerbated by being a menopausal Ph.D. student. She had treated me on a couple of occasions for electromagnetic stress but the results, though marvellous, were only temporary. Then she told me about The Procters. "Don't ask me how it works, just get in touch and ask if they can help you!" So I did.

'At the time I was working in an office with no natural light, no windows (except one looking out to a long internal corridor), and a doorway in each of the four walls; a reception area in fact. I remember my feeling on being told I had to work there — it was like being imprisoned. I even woke for a night or two after dreaming of being incarcerated in this small and poky environment. To cap it all, the space housed not only my desk and computer, but the office photocopier, fax and laser printing machines — all heavily used by several people throughout the day. The physical sensation when in the room was one of pressure on the head, a mild breathlessness (suffocation is perhaps not too

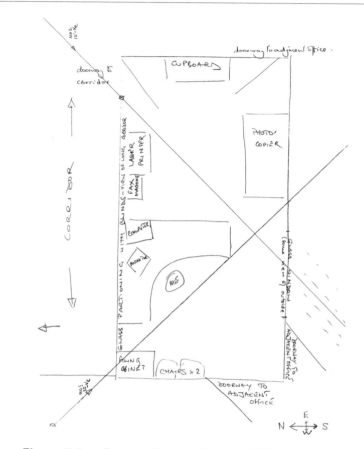

Figure 7.5 — Energy Lines at Diana's Office in Surrey

strong a word) and a *fizzing* feeling in my brain. This was
worse, of course, when the photocopier was being used.

'Discussions with a manager had led to the air conditioning
being improved. As far as I was concerned, this made a difference to the temperature but nothing else. This work had been
finished some five or six weeks before I contacted you with a
request to see what you could do to heal my home and working environments. (No-one else knew of this.) One Monday
morning, I walked into my office (with the usual sense of mixed
dread and resignation) to find that things felt rather different.
There wasn't time to analyse quite how and why as the usual

mass of work required immediate attention. However, after an hour or so, a male colleague walked through and commented on the difference in the atmosphere. 'The air conditioning must be working better — they probably altered something over the weekend.'

'I asked him what difference he noticed and he commented that the atmosphere was far lighter (it was too!) and generally more pleasant. We both agreed that we felt as if we had grown a few inches in height! At that time I had no knowledge that you had healed the building, but it was no surprise to find a letter on my return home on Tuesday evening saying that you'd worked on it over the weekend. The strangest thing was that someone who had no inkling of my contact with you, and who is not someone one would immediately think of as a sensitive soul (he is ex-army and somewhat gung-ho!), noticed the difference in atmosphere enough to comment upon it without any prompting at all.

'So there we are — a much happier and lighter environment in which to work — it really did improve matters hugely. Over the next few days, the sensation was of a cloud which had lifted, making everything (including the unpleasant physical symptoms) so much easier. As a final proof of the improved situation, Dr N. confirmed that the electromagnetic stress levels were almost zero.'

Vive les Procters!

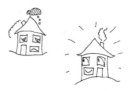

From Hugh in Devon

'I have always known in myself when entering a place or a building, if it seemed right. When I read last year an article in one of the Sunday supplements called "Home Sick Home" I felt the need to know more. I think the article was in *The Sunday*

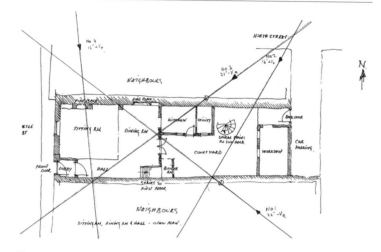

Figure 7.6 — Energy Lines at Hugh's House in Devon

Times which I rarely read, but we had friends staying who bought the paper. Fate playing its hand. Anyway, seeing your address at the bottom of the article after reading it, I wrote asking for more information. You sent me a series of leaflets about your Workshops. Workshop 1 being "Accessing your Intuition via Dowsing". So I booked and came on the first workshop, again, it felt *right*....

'I was a little nervous on the first visit, not knowing what to expect and what sort of people would come. I thought the discussions would be way above my head, and the conversations too high powered. I need not have worried. The first workshop I found fascinating, for instance, I was unaware that one can dowse just about anything if you ask the right questions. Finding out about the energy lines that criss-cross the planet; that they vary in polarity, width and strength. It was also interesting to see the many different ways of dowsing.

'After I left the first workshop I felt not only a sense of well-being but full of energy and a real sense of having enjoyed the day through meeting new people.

'Soon after that workshop we moved house. Before coming on the second workshop I let you know our new address. After attending the second workshop you informed me that our house had a couple of negative earth energy lines and would we like to have them changed. I sent a rough plan of the house to dowse, for you to address the negative energy lines.

'I felt our house was a *healthy* house before it was dowsed, but I did feel there was room for improvement. I had sensed that the previous owner of the house had not been entirely at ease when she had been living here. I have spoken with her subsequently and it would seem my feelings had been right. I did not find the negative lines oppressive in the house, maybe because my own energy was strong enough to counteract it. However, since altering the negative lines to positive the house does seem very relaxed and laid-back, if a house can be laid-back!'

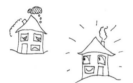

From Denny in Somerset
An Interview

Ann: 'We did some healing on your house. I haven't got the file out, but I remember that you had some quite amazing experiences at the other end.'

Denny: 'Let's start a little before I asked you. I moved into the property two or three days before and was sort of just getting used to it. It felt perfectly OK for the first couple of days, then I thought that there is something going on here that I don't particularly care for.'

Ann: 'How long ago was this that you moved in?'

Denny: 'Nineteen ninety-one, something like that, seven or eight years ago. So anyway, I got up on the Monday morning, I think, and was just going to brush my teeth when there was this almighty bang in my bedroom. I had a wonderful old glass vitrine with books in it which had blown itself across the room

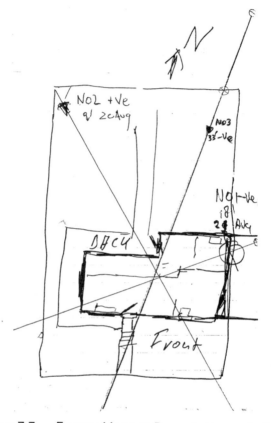

Figure 7.7 — Energy Lines at Denny's House in Somerset

a good ten or twelve feet. It had been high up on a wall and had gone to the other end of the room. I thought that this is not right! The glass was all shattered and smashed itself to smithereens. Pity, because it was a nice piece of furniture. So something was going on and needed to be checked out. As I was coming to you the next day for our regular healing group meeting, I thought that we could check it out then. I remember that we discovered two negative lines, I think, and healed them in the group session.'

Ann: 'I think so, yes.'

Denny: 'I decided to go back and experience this.'

Ann: 'The more fool you!'

Denny: 'I came home. It was quite turbulent. Then the house circuit breaker blew and would not reset despite removing fuses from various circuits to try to isolate the fault. None of this was any good as the breaker just would not stay in whatever I tried. So decided that it was now time to just go to bed! I remember very clearly lying in bed was like a bit of science fiction, or *Back to the Future*; a swirling time tunnel and I was travelling along at a fair rate of knots although perfectly awake and aware, for about half an hour or so. I wasn't hallucinating or under the influence of anything I had taken. And then 'it just began to quieten down. Now my bed was virtually over one of the lines, so I had experienced being inside a negative line changing to positive. The next morning everything was normal, the electricity was back and everything worked OK. That is the story.'

Ann: 'Yes, but there was another bit that I was thinking you were going to tell. We did another healing some time after that time, you had a friend in who was an expert in electrics, and the electrics went off again and he could not find anything wrong with it.'

Denny: 'Oh yes! that's right, there was a second round. You had done some healing remotely when I was at home some years later, and something went in the house; the electrics failed, and we could not find a fault. But after a while I remembered that I do have a surge detector to protect the television from power surges, lightning strikes etc., and that had been blown to bits, literally! The healing was so powerful!'

Ann: 'I am sorry, we didn't mean to do that. We just wanted to heal your line for you!'

Denny: 'Well it was the power surge protector blowing up that had caused all the rest to go.'

Ann: 'So when the healing was done, it was the power surge protector that blew up. And that upset everything else?'

Denny: 'Yes. It was so much power going through the house.'

Ann: 'Well I didn't know we could cause anything like that! Anyway, what happened after that? Did the energies feel better?'

Denny: 'Yes, it was fine after that.'

Ann: 'Did we do healing any more than on those two occasions?'

Denny: 'I don't think so. I have asked for you to check the lines again from time to time and I do not think you found anything more wrong. On those occasions it may have been more to do with me I would assume.'

Ann: 'Thank you, Denny. I am only sorry that your animated gestures and expressions won't come out on the tape! They made this little interview great fun! I have to say that your experience of electrical anomalies coincident with a healing of earth energies is unique! People often have reactions, but none so dramatic as you report.'

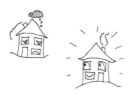

From Sarah in Wales

'In January of last year I forwarded a sketch plan of the floor area of my house so that you could rebalance the energies with dowsing.

'At the time, I felt that the house required healing. A church on the opposite side of the street had been demolished, and you agreed that this could have contributed to changing the quality of the energy lines.

'Although I did not contact you immediately following your dowsing, I'm sure you will be pleased to hear that I believe your work had a positive effect. I wrote to you on Monday, 4 January 1999. You had not indicated when you began working on my house, nonetheless, on Friday 8 January, on returning home, I was aware of a lightness, and even warmth. There had

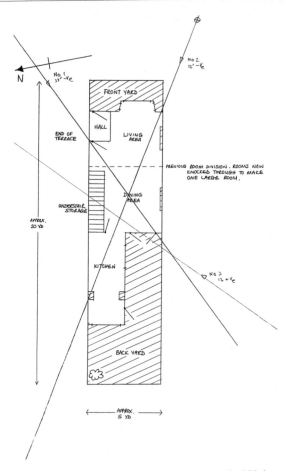

Figure 7.8 — Energy Lines at Sarah's House in Wales

previously been a feeling of weight. It was almost easier to breathe, and the continuous *muzzy* headache I had been experiencing for some time lifted over a few weeks. My husband, mother, and a number of visitors also remarked on how airy or bright the house felt, despite them not all being aware that I had contacted you.

'Given that any scepticism I may have initially felt has now been firmly allayed, I am writing to ask that you continue to keep my case under review for another twelve months. This is especially important at this time, as work began on 10 January 2000, to build a new church on the old site. The work is likely to continue for nine months, and I am aware it could result in changes in the positive energies that you have created.'

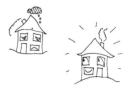

From Jane in East Sussex

'We moved to this house in May 1998, and felt it necessary to work on various levels to improve the energy flows inside and outside the house in order to help our work as therapists and healers. There was great improvement but we still didn't feel it was *right*. It took lots of energy and efforts to accomplish things and we were experiencing poor and broken sleep. We felt we needed some help to balance the remaining problems and we heard of Ann and Roy from other therapists so we sent off our map and donation.

'Their reply was waiting for us after we returned home from being away on a week's course. We were told that two negative ley lines had been changed to positive. Also since we thought there had been farm buildings on the site before the house was built, Ann and Roy checked for *entities* and *presences* left over from those times. In the past people buried an animal on the hearth or threshold as a guardian of the place. Ours was apparently not pleased with the new building and felt confused and unrespected. They had done some explaining and appeasing but it needed our respect too. They asked us to find a suitable article to place by the fireplace or by the front door and dedicate it to the guardian so that it had somewhere to reside in the house.

'The work on the ley lines had definitely created a much lighter feeling in the house. Initially we could not think of any article to give to the guardian and gradually over a week drifted by. Eventually one morning feeling the need to take some

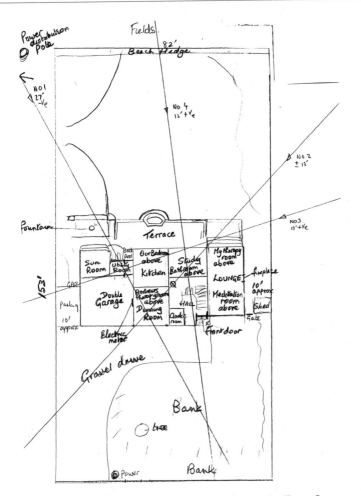

Figure 7.9 — Energy Lines at Jane's House in East Sussex

action, I moved a very large pebble I'd brought from the garden; and put it by the front door saying a few appropriate words to the guardian. I carried on with my working day forgetting to say anything to my husband.

'We both woke up the next morning rather surprised as we'd had the best night's sleep since we'd lived here. Some while later I remembered the pebble but decided still not to say anything to my husband. The following night we again slept so well that it prompted my husband to express his amazement. I then told him about the pebble.

'We have to say that our sleep patterns have remained much better. The energy in the house is calmer and clearer, more relaxed and we are accomplishing things with less effort.'

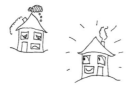

From Mrs L in Surrey
A Progression of Letters

10 June 1999: 'I feel very strange that I do not want to be here when I return from our caravan (tourer) holidays, which I love. I have always been a home-lover, but there seems to be an unknown atmosphere which makes me very depressed, although any visitors always say what a lovely atmosphere of calm there is here. I absolutely dread the winter when we cannot go away. We have lived here twenty-one years. My husband

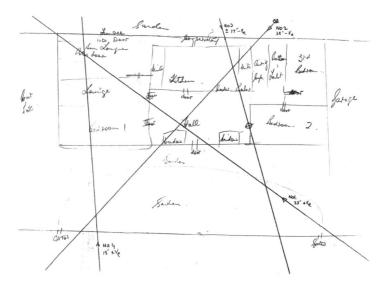

Figure 7.10 — Energy Lines at Mrs L's House in Surrey

is totally unaware of anything, he is seventy-nine and I am seventy-six this month.'

14 June 1999: Healing done.

October 1999: 'As a follow-up, as promised, I have found returning home from being in our caravan was not nearly as depressing as I found it previously. I normally dread the winter, but it seems a less daunting outlook this year. I am sure your help has made a difference and as, at the moment, I am recovering from a hip replacement, home is very welcome. I feel very guilty complaining about a lovely bungalow when so many have real cause to grumble.'

January 2000: 'I have found I have felt more settled since your *treatment*, but have not really noticed any improvement in my general health. I heard of your help through my homoeopathic doctor.'

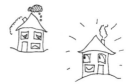

From Denise and Mike on the North Coast of Scotland

'We live in a beautiful part of the world. It's somewhat remote, bleak in bad weather, but glorious in the sunshine when we look across the Pentland Firth to the Orkney Islands; or climb down the grassy cliff at the back gate to walk along the beach, where seals swim inquisitively alongside and wading birds search along the sea's edge.

'Our family of four was fortunate in living a fairly carefree existence. I did notice, however, that if I sat for long in certain parts of the house I became really tired, and often very cold. This had been since we moved north fifteen years ago. My husband did not feel this — he never really feels cold, so I put it down to my circulation. Our children, now much further south, did not notice anything in particular.

'I was reading *The Sunday Times* supplement one weekend when I noticed an article on "Healing Sick Houses" — and something seemed to click. I wrote to Ann and Roy, who had been inundated with mail as a result of the article, and they replied asking me to send a ground map of the house indicating north. I sent this and also described the area because the article had given earth disturbance as one of the ways in which energies turn negative. We have sea and cliffs to the north, remains of Neolithic settlements on a nearby hill to the west, a new building (my mother's flat) to the east and a road to the south which serves the nearby harbour. Also, we had recently been put on mains drainage so there had been a lot of deep digging to the north end of the garden.

'I did not know when Ann and Roy were going to dowse, but one day I felt a subtle difference in the house. I phoned them to say things were feeling much better but I sensed there was still some negativity. They had asked for feedback to check how things were going. My sister was staying with me when the lines finally became positive. On the Tuesday she suddenly remarked how nice the house was feeling, and I told her I had been noticing this too. I phoned Ann and Roy the next evening, and they told me that on Monday night, with their dowsing group, they

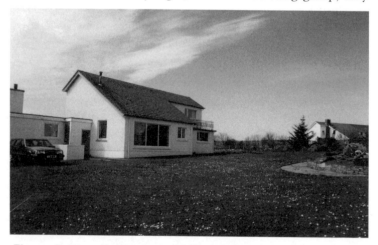

Figure 7.11 — Denise's and Mike's House

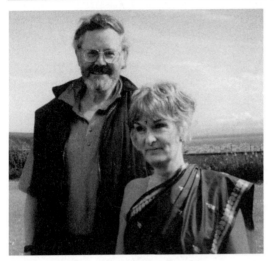

Figure 7.11a — Mike and Denise

had worked on the area rather than the house as one of the members specialised in healing sick areas.

'I've no idea what was the cause, but all I can say is that the house feels better and I don't get so tired and cold. My husband still does not notice any difference but says he's just an insensitive male! My sister certainly noticed the change when she was staying with us. We did not know when the Procters were working on the house or area and as we were both very busy we were not waiting and looking for something to happen. Another interesting point is that my energy levels seem much better now. The dragging feeling that used to slow me down almost to a point of stasis has gone — I have more energy to give to my business, which has taken an upward turn, and am back to being creative, directing a production of "A Midsummer Night's Dream" at our local theatre.

'I like to seek explanations for such things, but also keep an open mind, believing that humans have a lot more to discover and rediscover about ourselves and the world we live in! Because I work in the field of complementary health (nutrition and magnetotherapy) I do not think the changes I felt in myself were due to changes in my health. It is generally good — but

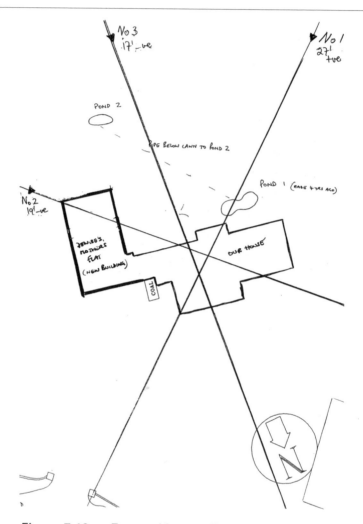

Figure 7.12 — Energy Lines at Denise's and Mike's House, on the North Coast of Scotland

the tiredness and coldness were apparent in certain areas of the house. Although I obviously get cold and tired sometimes, I don't now get the dragging sensations when sitting in a chair by the south-facing window in the living room, or on the settee on the north side as I used to. The house is always full of physical light with its large and many windows, but I now feel there is a different quality within the place. The best way I can describe it is to say it feels as though some heaviness has been taken away. In some way it was a sick house, and I am grateful to Ann and Roy and their group for healing it.'

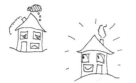

From Angela in Somerset

'I had consulted Ann Procter for some counselling help after completion of a course of chemotherapy which had left me total-ly drained and rather ill. I was rather surprised to get a commu-nication from her shortly after the first consultation: to the effect that my house was in pretty bad shape; and there was a *presence* in the house badly affected by an object, but that all could be put right by healing if I so wished.

'I had moved to the house from London about three years previously, and although intellectually I knew it was a good move and that the house was the right size etc. and really just what I had wanted, I had never really settled down properly. I

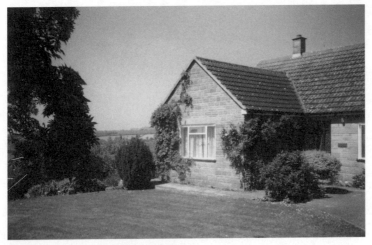

Figure 7.13 — Angela's House

was always asking myself whether I had been wise to move, and no matter how I tried to make the house my home, there was always something missing. The kitchen particularly, I felt did not welcome me properly. I therefore thought that healing the house might be a good thing, especially if the object was dealt with.

'After presenting a floor plan of the house, I was amazed to discover the extent and size of the negative lines that were running all over the place. Obviously my house must have been pretty sick!

'The healing accordingly took place, without my knowing anything about it at the time, and about four days later I began to feel a great deal more comfortable about the house in general. After another session with Roy and Ann, the undesirable object was dealt with, and as a result of all this activity the house is much more welcoming and I feel much more settled down here.

'It is very difficult to be positive about such a nebulous thing as a feeling about one's house, but I feel convinced that the healing has made a definite and very real contribution to the recovery of my spirits and energy over the past couple of months.'

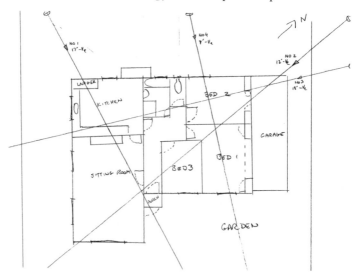

Figure 7.14 — Energy Lines at Angela's House in Somerset

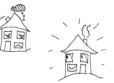

From S.T. in London NW6

'I work as an alternative health practitioner (mostly from my home) and use my spare room for therapy space. Despite having had my flat Feng Shui'd by a well-respected and experienced practitioner, I remained puzzled about why, despite all my efforts to increase my client list, it remained obstinately small and erratic and my financial status was therefore increasingly worrying. In addition, my energy was on the whole low and I had apparently developed an allergy to pollen, cats and house dust which gave me quite severe breathing problems from time to time.

'I did one of the Procters' workshops in the summer of 1999 and was very interested to learn that Roy and Ann had dowsed all the addresses of participants looking for negative energies. To my consternation, I was told there were some in my flat. My immediate thought was that this might explain some of my problems so I had no doubts about asking them to heal the space. The required ground plans of flat and garden were duly sent, along with a note that George, one of my cats, loved sitting on a particular spot on the garden wall. This turned out to be significant as it was where one of the energies entered my property. I wasn't entirely surprised to learn that two negative energies also crossed through my therapy space.

'I didn't know when the healing was going to be done but was aware of a dramatic change in my life one day not long after. The phone started ringing with clients wanting appointments, a general feeling of heaviness died and the cat started sitting in another part of the garden! A couple of days later, I received a letter from Ann informing me the healing had taken place. Immediately I rang them to tell them the differences I had noticed and to check when the healing had taken place.

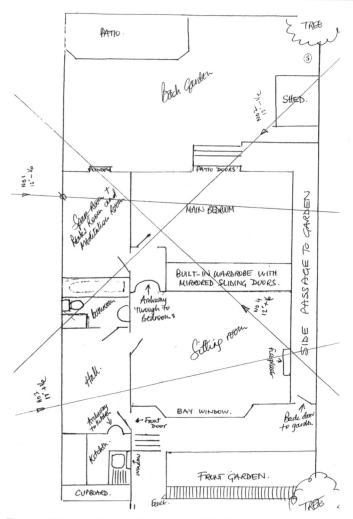

Figure 7.15 — Energy Lines at S.T.'s Flat in London NW6

It turned out it had been performed the day before I noticed the changes. Very interesting indeed!

'Sadly, the increase in business didn't continue so that is obviously down to other factors (although I'm sure the negative energies didn't help), so my financial situation is still dodgy. Of late, (three months after the healing) my health has improved and I am far less asthmatic which is very good news. The cat does still

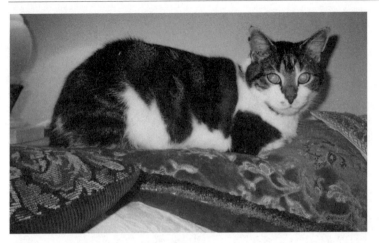

S.T.'s cat sitting in a new place.

sit on his old favourite spot sometimes, but mostly he seems to be trying out other places.

'Despite not experiencing a complete reversal of my situation, I am convinced that the healing has brought about positive and beneficial changes and I am very pleased I have had it done. I have recommended Ann and Roy to clients and friends and would have no hesitation in continuing to do so.'

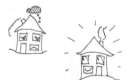

From Margaret in Gloucestershire

'I had lived in my 1690 house in Gloucestershire quite comfortably for many years, when it slowly became apparent that all was not well. I became increasingly tired, depressed, unable to sleep and felt the need to get away from my house, and I actually considered moving.

'Holidays were always enjoyed, but coming home quickly dispersed the light-heartedness I felt while away. I was not ill, (this was checked) but feelings continued of dullness, exhaustion and lack of energy.

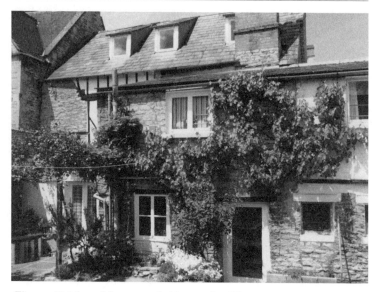

Figure 7.16 — Margaret's House in Gloucestershire

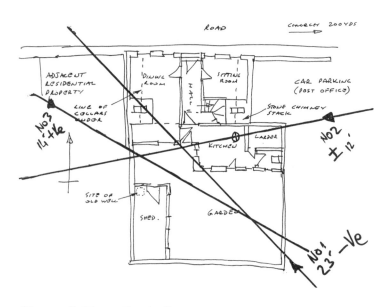

Figure 7.17 — Earth Energies at Margaret's House in Gloucestershire

'In an effort to boost my health I consulted a kinesiologist for advice and food supplements. After months of treatment the kinesiologist suggested that my house could be dragging me down and if so, geopathic stress was likely to be the cause. It was recommended that I contact Ann and Roy Procter for help.

'I did this and after some initial dowsing from their home of the earth energies at my house they discovered that of the three energy lines running through the house, two were negative. I asked Ann and Roy to heal these energies and they later reported that all the energies were now positive.

'I did not know exactly when the healing took place, but before I received Ann and Roy's confirming letter I had already noticed a change. I no longer had restless disturbed nights but benefited from deep refreshing sleeps that helped lift my spirits. I did not lose my drained feelings immediately but over the following months my tiredness eased and I became more focussed and clearer in my own mind about what I needed to do to move forward.

'Gradually my energy is returning and with it optimism and wellbeing. Most rewarding of all is the relaxed harmonious atmosphere now prevalent in my home.'

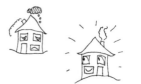

From Fion in Northampton

'I have no doubt that changes for the better are already occurring for me and my son. We are both so much more relaxed in the house — both much less living on our nerves and having a better time all round. It is a joy to look at my little boy's face and see that the jumpy tension that has been there as long as I can remember has gone. Yesterday he started talking about being a star spirit after he dies and how he wants to travel through outer space before being born again! Tonight he said that the

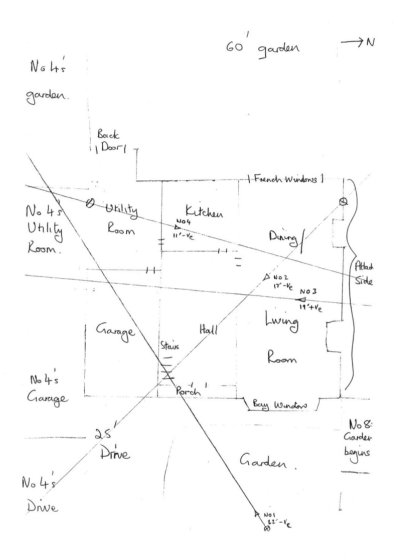

60' garden   → N

No 4's
garden.

Back
Door

French Windows

No 4's
Utility
Room.

Utility
Room

Kitchen

No 4
11'-ve

Dining

Attad
Side

No 2
17'-ve   No 3
          11'+ve

Garage

Hall

Living

Room

No 4's
Garage

Stairs

Porch

Bay Window

No 8:
Garden
begins

25'
Drive

Garden.

No 4's
Drive

No 1
22'-ve

Figure 7.18 — Earth Energies at Fion's House in Northampton

wonderful thing about having his own special angel was that his
angel will always be with him. It is quite a while since he talked
like that (he's just five) and it's lovely to hear it again.

'I was very interested (and reassured) at what you wrote about a guardian here. Any dwelling here would have had to have been built in the 1600s or before from what I understand of local history.

'Last night I did a small ceremony: lighting a candle, honouring the guardian, apologising for the disruption to it and assuring it of a welcome here in a place of its own. What I saw and felt was a badger sett and then the bodies of two badgers, left together, buried in the sett.

'Either side of my fireplace are two small recesses and so I have put a small black stone in one and a small white stone in the other as an acknowledgement of their welcome and place here. It feels right and I feel very honoured to have a guardian presence in my home and at my hearth.'

Chapter 8

WHAT CAN *YOU* DO?

We all do a lot, all the time, to design and influence the atmosphere of our homes, or other places where we spend our time. This matters a lot more for some people than for others. Are you happy to live in an untidy tip not likely to pass hygiene inspections, or do you want everything spick and span and squeaky clean in order to feel comfortable? When you go into someone else's house, particularly if you are house-hunting and thinking of living in that place yourself, do you notice shapes of rooms, colours, views through windows and orientation (i.e. which way will the sun come in)? Do you get a subtle *feel* for the place? On a number of occasions we have been asked to dowse, and subsequently heal, a house which is on the market, welcoming viewers but getting no offers. Are the visitors only dismissing the room layouts or the state of the brickwork, or are they unconsciously sensing something not right with the place? We never offer any guarantees, but our experience is that potential buyers do warm to a house with positive earth energies. In one case someone paid cash for a place the day after we healed it: it had been on the market for a year!

So can you *cure* your own sick house? Up to a point, yes, but if there are negative earth energies running through it, probably not. Doing the diagnostic part of it by dowsing would require a very high degree of detachment: you are likely to be too involved in what you are going to find to get truly intuitive answers to your questions — the emotional and instinctive levels will be in full force, concerned about the state of your nest. On the few occasions when we have been concerned about the state of our energy lines here at home, we have found it prudent to ask a colleague to dowse, and, if necessary, heal for us.

Human Effects

Here are some reasons why your energy lines might go negative. We have noticed that if something with a particularly strong impact happens on an energy line, especially if on its centre, the polarity reverses from there on down the line depending on which direction it is flowing. So choose to have your rows somewhere else! This reversal has been known to happen where someone dies, or has some bad news — it's the magnitude of emotional experience which seems to have the effect. An example of this came to light recently when a client mentioned that she had been dismayed to find that a house was being built near her boundary, taking away the nice view she had had from her kitchen sink: every time she stood there she felt very sad and that spot had become negative. Outside your control are major earthworks etc., but people who notice such excavations happening near their homes sometimes ask us to check if their lines are still positive. Certainly it's worth checking if you have an extension or something built, requiring digging down for foundations.

Feng Shui

The interactions between humans, the animal and plant kingdoms and the subtle environment have been known since ancient times. Perhaps the best known system is Feng Shui, which is a discipline of manipulating the subtle environment from ancient China. As practised in the West, Feng Shui seems mainly concerned with the interior of buildings and the types and placement of furniture and colours. Whether this is effective or not no doubt depends on the practitioner and the power of intention over and above the practical advice. Our feeling is that in-house Feng Shui can be beneficial but is not the whole solution. We think that the underlying earth energies must also be harmonised and this will often be due to matters well outside the building itself. In fact, we have found agreement in this from some Feng Shui practitioners who have attended our courses in order to complement their skills by dealing with the earth energies as well. Some also refer their clients to us for healing before doing their own work.

A Suitable Healing Base

If you are doing healing work of any kind, it is even more important that you have the *right* place to do it in. We think that the qualities of the place where healing is carried out is important for good results. We usually do all our work in Ann's study/consulting room which has a very good atmosphere. One of the reasons that we came to live in this house is because of the very powerful and beneficial earth energy lines running through the house and grounds.

We had an interesting lesson about this a couple of years ago. As a result of an article that gave our work some publicity, we had many enquiries. Although we had tried to clear this work up to date before going on holiday in Scotland, we still had a few cases waiting to be done by the day of departure. So, as we were going to a beautiful place on the Isle of Mull in our caravan, we decided to take the file with us and do the healing work as part of one of our morning meditations.

After a long two-day journey with the caravan we arrived at the site late on the second day, put down the steadies on the van, had a meal and retired to bed. Ann did not sleep well. The next morning she wondered if we had parked the van in the wrong place. We usually dowse for the earth energy qualities when we stop in our caravan before settling down. Due to lateness and tiredness the night before, we had not done this. We now found that there was a small negative spot under the van, in fact under Ann's side of the bed. Needless to say we moved the van a few feet into a clear space before finally setting up the awning etc. Good sleep was had for the rest of the holiday.

A day or so later, when we had sufficiently recovered from the journey, we decided to tackle some of the healing work.

Starting dowsing with the usual check questions we soon established that it was inappropriate to continue. This seemed to be because we were in the wrong place for this work. This tended to confirm our belief that when doing this type of healing, not only are we calling down help from higher powers above, but that we also need to tap into the earth energy system at an appropriate point. Our caravan was no longer on a bad place. It was just that it was not on a good enough place for this work. Thus, we believe that therapists of all kinds, and particularly alternative ones who work largely on an intuitive basis moving energies, should look into the earth energy qualities of their healing place.

A Note for Healing Therapists

We have come to recognise that healing activity can easily leave some residues lying around, to the detriment of the subtle energies of the place where the healing happened. This discovery started when we were taking part in a week-long event on Iona, working with doctors and healers in the Abbey complex. One of the participants, whom we had met as fellow students of Bruce MacManaway, told us he had dowsed a black stream (his term for a negative earth energy line) in the Abbey Church and he wanted us to help him heal it. We said we would not do anything without the permission of the Iona Community, which manages the precinct, and anyway, in such a place there could well be some reason for this phenomenon; so we advised watching and waiting. Sure enough, at the evening healing service, Ann perceived that, as people received healing and felt better, they dropped something of their troubles, and this negative stuff disappeared into the black stream our friend had found. It was as if it needed a sink or plughole to dispose of it into the earth, leaving the church clean and light. When increasing the light, something has to be done to let the dark move on. As we did not have a ready-made subtle sink in our healing room at home, we designated one by keeping a bowl of water on the windowsill, emptying it with intent into a negative spot in the garden after a healing session.

We found thereafter that we were rarely affected by the troubles, pains and miseries of our clients, whether they had asked us for healing personally or for their home, or for Ann's professional work in psychotherapy and counselling. So since then we have recommended to a number of centres where healing takes place — at any level, including in doctors' surgeries — that they have a disposal system of some kind. It's not the method by which it's done that matters, it's the intent the healer puts into it which makes it work, so we have heard of several other rituals which are working well. We have had a considerable amount of feedback about the efficacy of this system, particularly from people at the Bristol Cancer Help Centre, where Ann worked for seven years. They did not know we had placed a bucket of water in the basement to collect the dross, but they noticed the change in atmosphere! Before the bucket was installed someone had said it felt 'like the psychic drains backing up'. A healer meditating in the sanctuary (where a great deal of spiritual healing is given) remarked one day that the room was 'as black as your hat': we found that the bucket had been removed by heating engineers attending to the boiler! Before starting this ritual it was difficult to keep the earth energy lines in this large building in a positive state; it seemed that the backwash of so much healing activity strained the earth energies so much that they turned negative after a while. This did not happen once the bucket ritual was being maintained because there was an appropriate disposal channel.

Electric and Electromagnetic Effects

When we are dowsing for subtle aspects in the environment for people (*see* Chapter 4 and Appendix 2) we often find they are being affected by, for one thing, domestic electricity. We learned about this from a colleague who was very severely affected, unable to work and having difficulty looking after her small son. Her husband, a scientist, set up all kinds of experiments to see if he could alleviate her suffering. They covered every electrical socket in the house with aluminium foil, and at one stage the lady was wearing a straw hat, come rain or shine, lined with foil! Eventually they found that if a cluster crystal is placed on the fuse box, or wherever the mains electricity cable comes into the house, the harmful effects are cancelled out. So if we find that is a problem for any of our clients, that measure is what we suggest. An architect pointed out to us that in this country we usually arrange our electrical circuits in the form of ring mains, which means we are surrounded by the electrical current in every room. He told us that in Germany this is forbidden: all electrical supplies are on spurs, so that they do not surround you.

A cluster crystal is a lump of natural crystal (not lead crystal) with lots of points, not a single bar. Quite a small one — one to three inches across (and one can dowse for the size, or select one in a shop by dowsing) will suffice. Amethysts are usually cheapest for size, but it does not matter what kind of crystal it is, so long as it has plenty of surface area. We learned the reason for this from Alan Hall, whose work we mentioned in Chapter 1: natural crystals have a minute layer of water all over their surface, only a molecule thick. This water picks up the electrical and electromagnetic vibrations that some people find detrimental. So we advise regular cleansing of the crystals placed for this purpose: under running water is usually enough, but sometimes a spring clean of all four elements would be helpful. We put ours out in the garden when we go on holiday so that they experience earth (on which they rest), fire (from the sun), air (as it passes by) and water (when it rains).

In some cases we dowse effects from microwaves beaming toward peoples' homes from communication discs, aerials etc., which now proliferate in our environment. Other people need protection from microwave emanations and cathode ray tubes in the home. If we dowse that clients are being depleted by these we suggest crystals placed on or very near TV sets and computer screens on the same basis as for the electrical effects above. In the case of beams from outside, we suggest a crystal on the point where it enters the house: we dowse for this position, which is often very precise. When we mention microwaves people often think we mean ovens, but their effect is usually on the food cooked in them, not on their immediate surroundings.

So, if you feel that electrical or electromagnetic factors may be part of any depletions you are feeling, it could be worth trying these measures, even if no-one has dowsed them for you. The small crystals suggested are not expensive (£5 or less) and they do look good as ornaments anyway.

You may notice that our checklist (Appendix 2) includes airborne pollution; we added this because someone eventually reported that a gas leak was the cause of their ill health, and we hadn't spotted it. This is a disadvantage of not visiting a house, as we would expect Ann to detect it physically: she only has half her lungs, and any air pollution affects her like a canary down a coal mine! (In case you haven't heard about that, it's a true story that if coal miners suspected foul air they took a canary down with them. If they were right, the canary rapidly took sick.) On one or two occasions we have discovered a problem with Radon gas, and can advise the client to take up the testing arrangements that are provided by the government.

A Dowsing Lesson

Having suggested that you do not attempt to diagnose earth energies in your own home, we would not like to discourage you from trying dowsing for yourself. You may like to follow this brief dowsing lesson, so that you can experiment with the skill in a general way. We have to say that it is difficult to learn this skill just from reading about it — you really do need hands-on practice and help from someone who is experienced in dowsing.

In our courses we introduce students to dowsing with the pendulum initially. This is because it is the most versatile tool and enables all the essentials of dowsing to be comprehended. The pendulum we advocate for beginners is a simple lightweight plastic conical affair. Its lightness means that it responds quickly, so progress can be rapid. The length of the string is also important as this is related to the weight: light weight, short string; heavy weight, longer string. Our plastic pendulum weighs about four or five grams and the string is eight centimetres long to the knot. By holding the knot the length of string used is always the same so that one gets used to its particular characteristics. Any variations from the normal will be more obvious. When practised, a minor change in response may provide an important clue.

Try sitting quietly holding your hands in front of you, palms facing each other, and move them together and apart slowly; maybe with your eyes shut? Many people sense some slight force between the hands. This may be like a magnetic attraction or a resistance. Some describe the feeling as gently pressing on a party balloon. The existence of a sensation, which is very subtle, indicates that there is a difference between the two sides of the body, a polarity. When dowsing with a pendulum, one needs to be aware of this.

There are two schools of thought in interpreting the response from a pendulum. One says that such and such a motion means *yes* and another means *no*. We prefer that people find out their own responses, as individuals differ greatly. To do this, follow the procedures below.

Sit comfortably in an upright position. Hold the pendulum in the hand you write with (usually the right so we will assume this; if you are left-handed, reverse the following instructions). The string should be held lightly between thumb and forefinger with these digits pointing downwards and the wrist relaxed. Without crossing arms or legs, dangle the pendulum over the right knee. Initiate a swing of the pendulum backwards and forwards, then wait to see how the swing develops and note any pattern. Then, without moving any other parts of your body, move your right hand with the pendulum over the left knee, initiate a swing and note any developing pattern. The swing may rotate one way over one knee and the opposite way over the other. This is not always so. In Roy's case the swing continues back and forth on the right but goes from side to side on the left.

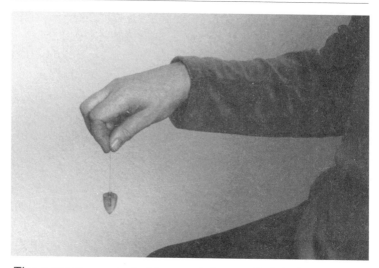

The correct way to hold a pendulum — lightly between thumb and forefinger with the hand and wrist as relaxed as possible.

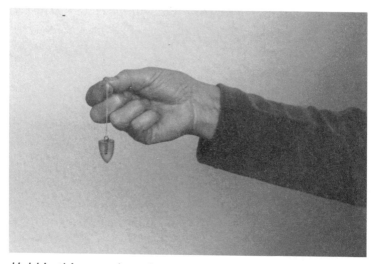

Held in this way there is more tension in the hand and muscles and less freedom for the fingers and thumb to help operate the pendulum.

Figure 8.1 — The Pendulum and How to Use It

When dowsing, **always** use the same hand in position on the same side of the body. The pattern when over your right knee will be your *yes* response and the one over your left knee during the above experiment will be your *no* response. When asking questions, however, remember to keep your dowsing hand in the same position all the time, otherwise your responses may change and totally confuse you!

Another way to find your own responses is to keep the hand over the right knee all the time. Give the pendulum a swing to get it started with some momentum, and ask, out loud if you like, for a *yes* response. Stop the movement by resting the pendulum briefly on your knee, then free and swing it again and ask for a *no* response. The different responses may be quite weak initially, but they will become stronger with practice.

Now, assuming that you have two different responses, you can begin to make use of the pendulum. Questions are posed (in the mind or out loud if that helps), the pendulum swung and the response noted. The pendulum can only signal *yes* or *no*, therefore questions must be carefully and unambiguously framed so that the answer is clear.

Before starting a series of questions it is important to make a few checks.

1. Check your responses. Ask for a *yes* response and a *no* response. See if they are what you are used to. Responses can change and if you have not checked this, you can get in a right muddle! Recheck responses from time to time during your dowsing session.
2. Ask, 'Am I fit to dowse **now**?' If you are very tired, had some alcohol or other drugs, are low in health or too emotionally involved, then you may not get accurate results. If the answer to this question is 'no', stop right then. There is no point in persisting or asking why, as the results are likely to be in error anyway. Try again later, particularly if you have time for a short meditation in order to centre yourself.

3. Ask, 'May we talk about...?' (Whatever the subject might be.)
   If the answer is 'no', go no further. It may be that the subject
   is not one that it is appropriate for you to look into. This rais-
   es the whole subject of ethics. Dowsing will only enable you
   to access information that it is suitable for you to know. It
   may be that a question on this particular matter cannot be
   answered at that time. Leave it, and try again later.

We cannot stress too much the importance of practice.
Confidence and accuracy only come from a great deal of practice. One of the difficulties is how to have meaningful practice.
Trying to dowse the numbers on a playing card randomly chosen will probably not give encouraging results. Finding such
numbers may be considered a pointless activity, so dowsing
doesn't work too well. Dowsing seems to need to be applied to
something *real* to be effective.

One exercise we have tried has the dowser work with another person and ask them about their front door. (This must be one
the dowser hasn't seen.) After the preliminary checks, the dowser asks a question such as, 'Is the door painted?' If 'yes' then try
some colours. 'Is the door green?' 'Is the door red?' 'Is the door
blue?' and so on. Each question should be posed out loud so
your assistant knows what you asked. You then say what the
dowsed answer is. Your assistant should just say 'right' or
'wrong' as the case may be, but not give the correct answer. The
point of this exercise is that you get instant feedback. Your assistant can also help by commenting on your questions. Clarity and
lack of ambiguity are most important. For instance, you may
have established that the door was made of wood but was not
painted; so you conclude that it is unpainted bare wood. It might
be varnished or stained, but you didn't ask. You made an invalid
assumption based on insufficient data!

Of course this game does not only have to be played with
front doors. Any subject you are unfamiliar with that your assistant knows about will do. We find that the most frequent source
of error in dowsing is in the question being unclear and/or

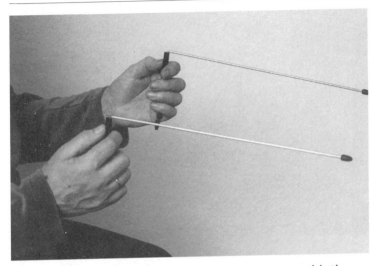

Rods should be held lightly — free to swing — with the tips slightly lower than the bend while searching, and about shoulder-width apart.

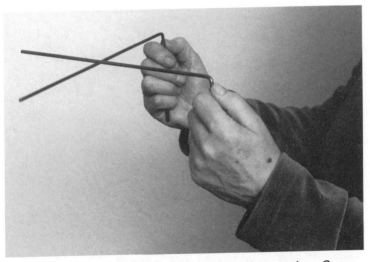

A dowsing reaction is usually by the rods crossing. Some may get the opposite — the rods opening away from each other.

Figure 8.2 — L-Rods and How to Use Them

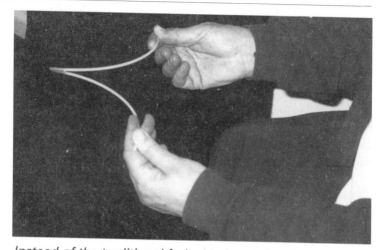

Instead of the traditional forked twig modern Y-rods are made of plastic because they are more springy and consistent. Shown is the correct method of holding while searching. The rods should be held curved and under tension.

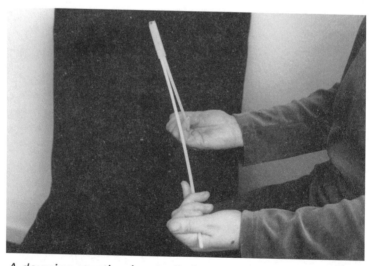

A dowsing reaction is usually by a dipping of the tip, but some people may find the tip flips up instead. (Mind your glasses!)

Figure 8.3 — Y-Rods and How to Use Them

ambiguous. This exercise is a great help in developing clarity. The assistant needs to be quite critical in checking your questioning process. When playing this game, be sure to maintain yourself in the correct dowsing position. If your assistant is sitting on your left, it is very easy to get engrossed in the questioning and gradually turn toward the other person to face them. The responses stop making sense. Then you notice that you have moved so that your right (pendulum) hand is positioned over your left side. The result is that your responses have changed as you are now *crossed*. No wonder confusion has set in!

So far we have only discussed the pendulum. Some people have difficulty initially in getting a response from a pendulum. In these cases we move outside and try them with L-rods.

These are held with the long end forwards, one in each hand at about shoulder-width apart. The tips of the rods should be very slightly lower than the handle end. The rods should be held loosely so that they are free to swing from side to side. We lay a piece of rope or something across the lawn and ask people to walk across it while asking the rods, 'Please indicate when I cross the rope'. Hopefully the rods will cross as you do so. This exercise helps get the sensation of a reaction from the rods from crossing a known line. So the exercise can be repeated over say, a buried water pipe. The reaction sensation can now be recognised more easily. The same experiment can be tried with Y-rods (*see* Chapter 4).

Relaxed muscles in shoulders give the rods a better chance of moving, as does a relaxed attitude. We find that distracting people or making them laugh often brings results, as it is all too easy to try too hard. Those who did not get on well with a pendulum initially often find results with the rods better because they involve moving about. Having cracked it they can usually return to the pendulum successfully.

Another tool very popular with dowsers is a bobber. This is a piece of springy material, usually wire, with a handle at one end and a small weight at the other end. It behaves like a

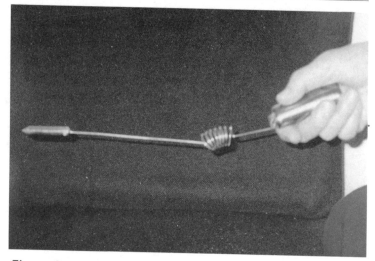

Figure 8.4 — A Bobber

horizontal pendulum, giving one signal for yes and another for no.

Nearly everyone can dowse. So if you are finding it difficult to get started, what might be the problem?

The dowsing reaction is often inhibited by tense muscles, because it is an unconscious small muscular movement of some sort. The dowsing tool used only serves to magnify these small involuntary movements so that they are obvious and easy to interpret. If the relevant muscles are already in a state of tension, then the small involuntary movements are masked and nothing shows. So posture is important. Sit or stand upright, don't slouch. The arm holding the pendulum should be as relaxed as possible with the upper arm hanging down and the forearm horizontal. The wrist should be relaxed with the thumb and forefinger pointing down and with a light grip on the string. Ensure that the arm is free and that the elbow is not resting on a knee or tight against the body. Tension shows even more readily when using dowsing rods; dropping shoulders releases it and allows the tools to work.

Some dowsers think that the material of the pendulum is important, that it should be a crystal or some other special material. This is not so; anything suitable will do. A piece of Blu-Tack on some cotton, an old nut on a piece of string. The weight and length of string are the important matters so that the swing *feels comfortable*. The timekeeping accuracy of a clock is not affected by the material of the hands on the face. Matchsticks jammed on the shafts will be just as good at telling the time as beautifully crafted brass hands. It is the mechanism that provides the accuracy. In dowsing, the tool is like the hands on the clock. You yourself are the mechanism! However, if you fancy working with a beautifully turned and polished wood pendulum, or whatever, that's fine too.

Thinking that you can't dowse definitely makes success more difficult! In the 1970s we attended many lectures and other events with the Wrekin Trust and other organisations. We were both trying to understand more about these subtle processes over a wide range of subjects. During one event an old gentleman showed Roy that he could obtain sensible dowsing responses from a pendulum. Ann could already do this, but Roy did not think this was the sort of thing chaps like him did, so he was astonished to find his previous assumption blown away. Like so many people he had been conditioned by education and society to consider only the logical and material aspects of life. It seemed to him that this new attribute of accessing his intuition was important, even sacred, and not to be abused. The questions he asked of himself were, 'Why have I been shown this? What am I supposed to do with it?' It was another five years before he found out. The experience now being gathered changed his whole outlook on life. What a pity it came in his late forties rather than earlier! However, the logical thinking and precision needed for his career in aeronautical engineering, his various constructive hobbies and his piloting of many different kinds of aircraft, did mean that his skills in clarity and focussing were most useful when he moved on to working on healing sick houses.

For Roy, dowsing provided the connecting link that made it possible for the intellectual engineer in him to explore the subtle worlds to some degree. Things were never the same again, as a whole new way of looking at the meaning of life opened up. One outcome was that we started to teach dowsing to others. Ann had been running classes and groups of various kinds since 1960, always wanting to share the contents of her 'toolbox' of skills wherever there was a need. So when we were asked to teach dowsing, initially by the College of Psychic Studies, it was easy to fall into that task. Now that it is a double act we hope that our joint approach makes it more interesting and lively for our students.

We moved to Somerset in 1984 and these courses now take up a lot of our time each summer. We both feel that teaching dowsing is a good and valuable way to help the modern materialist look into other information processes and the subtle worlds.

Happy dowsing!

Chapter 9

OTHER CONSIDERATIONS

There are a number of considerations to take into account when doing this kind of work. It really must be done with integrity, what many people would call 'professionally', valuing ethical aspects and respecting individuals. This means caring for each case, because it is of great concern to the person requesting help. It also means applying our best skills and attention and communicating adequately. The correspondence and phone calls often take longer than the dowsing and healing! If being professional means charging big fees, we are not in that ball game. It is customary for spiritual healers to ask for reasonable donations rather than set a fee, and we find that a satisfactory way of working. Those who are really pushed for funds can send us a little — we do think that some exchange is necessary — and those who can afford more can make up for the smaller amounts. We don't get rich, but feel our service is valued in practical terms.

Confidentiality and Permission

Another important aspect to consider is the ethical one of confidentiality. Dowsing enables one to access all sorts of information. Is it right to pry into other people's business without their permission? The answer is a clear *no*, otherwise it would be like looking into another's diary without asking first. A testing example might be a request to locate a lost person. Perhaps the lost person does not wish to be found. Suppose it was a husband who had left home and was living with another woman. He would not be best pleased to be found by a dowser! Our very few excursions into this field have been limited to a child who had run away from home, and a young woman with learning difficulties who had been seen getting into a car with a strange man. In fact, our dowsing for location did not help much, but in both cases the girls were located while we were focussing on them; which seems, from the healers' point of view, to be much more appropriate. No healing can happen, as we understand it, unless it is right in the total scheme of things — i.e. unless Upstairs gives it the nod. Similarly, we will not dowse regarding the health of a person, or the energies of their house, unless we first have their permission.

Space and Time

We have occasionally been asked to dowse for missing animals, and feel this is ethical but not likely to succeed, because unless they are stuck down a rabbit hole they are likely to move before the owner can get to the place we have designated. One way out of this would be to dowse for where the animal will be when it is found. But now we have to consider whether it is ethical to dowse for something in the future. Although dowsing takes us into a more timeless sphere of existence (*see* below), there are always several possibilities for future events, depending on what people do in the meantime: it's a concern about fate and free will. You might dowse for something to happen in the future, for instance, that someone will arrive at your house at a certain time. Then they have a puncture or get lost, after you have announced your dowsed findings; so they arrive later and you are shown to be wrong. We have even had a man ring up wanting to come to a dowsing course so that he could predict which horses would win races: he thought he would be able to make a killing with the bookmakers! We declined to teach him, as we considered this very unethical.

Dowsing, as we see it, is a sacred skill; and not to be used for personal gain over and above reasonable recompense for the training, time and skill involved. When dowsing, it is vital to remember that we are extending into an area of consciousness where time and space are much less finite. Being deliberately, for this purpose, less focussed in everyday space awareness, we can detect things that are happening at some considerable distance — hence our practice of dowsing and healing remotely. It saves a lot of time, energy and fuel! But it does mean that we need to take great care to define the space we are looking into: incomplete addresses and vague maps are inadequate for our purpose, although we find that Upstairs does not require a post code.

Slipping out of normal time is perhaps more insidious. We often have subjective experiences of time anomalies: 'time stood still', 'it seemed like ages', 'the event happened in a flash'. So don't expect your clock to keep you in a finite structure!

Checking that what we are detecting or doing is, or should be, happening now is a vital part of our dowsing questioning. This lesson was brought home to us one cold Easter, long before we started our own groups and Ann used to belong to a healing group at a house called The Priory near our Surrey home. During our opening meditation one of the group often did some automatic writing, producing messages which seemed to come from the monks who had lived there in the past. It was behind an old church and the supposition that the monks were communicating seemed reasonable — at least a workable hypothesis.

One day as we were gathering the lady of the house told us how she would like to convert some outbuildings into a centre for complementary health practitioners: nowadays there are such places in every other street, but then it was very unusual. The little matter of funding was holding her back. To our surprise the writing gave us news that the monks had hidden treasure in the yard at the back of the house, so she could use that for her project. One member managed to borrow a metal detector, which didn't work, so the Procters were asked to try dowsing. Ann drew a diagram of the cobbled yard on squared paper, and brought it home. We dowsed for an exact position, and a depth, and in order to know what we were looking for, we asked about the kind of container the treasure was in (metal, wood, cloth etc.) and got ceramic. On Good Friday we duly took out some cobbles and dug down 2'3" in the spot dowsed. There was nothing, only some bits of broken brick among the disturbed earth, so, as it got darker and colder, we went home.

Next morning we returned to find that some joker had put a house brick painted gold in the hole! We investigated further and found, nearer to the house as well as further into the yard from our hole, a conduit made of small thin bricks set in a square, such as was used to form a drainpipe for very old houses. The little bricks were whole versions of the pieces we had found in the debris. So...? Ann did not mention the unfound treasure when the group next met, she was too embarrassed! But the writing gave us, in monkish language, 'Hard luck, we put it there, someone must have pinched it since.' We shall never know, but it seems as if we found the right place, but we had not asked if the treasure was there **now**. Anyway, it was enough to teach us the lesson, which is what mattered. Years later Roy had a couple of experiences emphasising our ability to get outside *normal* time:

'I used to work at Westland Helicopters in Yeovil. I also worked sometimes for one of their associated companies and had an office in London too. It was winter and I was leaving the Yeovil works in the dark, in my car. Near the works exit is a roundabout which I usually went across and continued straight on. There is then about three miles of road with only a single turning off before the next roundabout. This is the junction with the main A303 road and I usually turned right onto the A303 for home there. On this night there was conflicting traffic on the first roundabout, so I stopped and waited for a clear space. Continuing round the roundabout I turned off left at the usual exit but immediately became confused. Instead of the road being long and straight, it swung to the right and I did not recognise it at all. My immediate thought was that I had taken the wrong exit from the roundabout. But I knew those roads well and this was not one of them! I proceeded slowly on and in a few yards found myself in some sort of parking area with signs of construction about to begin.

'Still baffled, I got out of the car to have a look round with no idea as to where I was. Looking over the hedge where there was traffic, I saw a green road sign showing London to the left and Exeter to the right. So I got back into the car, turned round and started back round the curve the way I came and found myself at a roundabout on the A303 and turned toward London. I immediately recognised the road as my usual one away from the second roundabout. So it appeared that I had entered the first roundabout and completed the manoeuvre by exiting the second one with no intervening section!

'This transition was absolutely seamless. I was certainly fully wide awake and concentrating on the driving amid dense traffic. What is the explanation? The easy one is that my mind had wandered on to other matters (as one does sometimes) and had just not registered driving along the three-mile interconnecting road between the two roundabouts. This is certainly not the case as I had the car radio on all the time, tuned to Radio 4. Just as I was leaving the factory the PM programme finished and the shipping forecast started. This fixed the time at 5.50 p.m. exactly. As I was driving away from the second roundabout on the A303, the shipping ended and the general weather forecast started. This established the time at 5.55 p.m. exactly. Thus, five minutes had elapsed for the journey between the factory and onto the A303. This is too short. While going back and forth over the next few days I carried a stopwatch and timed the journey between these two points. It was generally about eight minutes and forty seconds. It also usually took between three and four minutes to drive between the two roundabouts. So there seems to be about three or four minutes missing out of my life in which I moved instantaneously a distance of a bit under three miles. Very odd and I have no logical explanation.

'Some months later I was in the London office. We occupied two floors and my office was one of a suite on the lower floor accessed through swing doors off the lobby. One day I was on my way to the cashier's office on the floor above. As I was about to go through the swing doors, a colleague was coming in the

opposite direction in a hurry. I held the doors open to let him
whizz through and continued up the stairs, along the corridor
and into the cashier's office. Imagine my surprise to find the
same colleague sitting at the cashier's desk writing out a cheque
for her! He had not passed me on the direct route to the cashier's
office and I had not stopped off on the way. I asked him how
long he had been there. 'Oh, a few minutes,' he said. He agreed
that he had not seen me on the way up. So this short walk
seemed to have taken some minutes longer than it should and I
was apparently absent for some of it. Again, from my perspective, it was totally seamless with no apparent discontinuities.

'Explanation? I don't have one: but it does make one wonder
about concepts of time and space. I also wonder if the missing
time from the first event is the same as the added time of the second!'

Protection

Another important aspect is that of protection of the dowser.
When dowsing one is *looking into* another state of existence,
sphere of information or whatever you like to call it. It is a different system with its own rules and they are not necessarily the
rules that we regard as normal. There are other energies and
intelligences in that system that are not always benign. So it is
important that the dowser retains a focus on goodness and rightness at all times. This is to prevent any influence or attachments
of a negative sense from affecting the dowser. We find that we
need to still our minds, focus on the *light* and ask permission to
look into the subject matter before proceeding.

It sometimes happens that dowsing responses can be giving
conflicting or confusing signals. This we call interference and it
may be compared to interference on the radio. Radio signals can
be of poor quality due to atmospheric problems or the programme may be distorted because someone is deliberately jamming the station. Similar situations can occur when dowsing. The
solution is usually to stop, recentre oneself, and then try again.
It may even be prudent to stop the session altogether and try

again another day. This may be particularly relevant if the dowser is somewhat tired or has been working too long in one session. We usually find that an hour to an hour and a half for one
of our dowsing and healing sessions is as much as we can manage with confidence, and it was a great deal less when we were
less experienced.

There are at least two good books on psychic protection (*see*
Bibliography and References, Section 7). The best means are
those devised by the individual to suit themselves, because the
necessary impetus comes from within the psyche and is always
unique. Some common ones are variations on imagining putting
oneself in light in some form. When she was little, our elder
daughter had night terrors, which meant we were often disturbed in the night. Eventually, when she was three or four, she
managed to learn to put herself in 'an eggshell of light', and we
all slept a lot better thereafter. For people who understand and
work with the human subtle energy system, the aura, filling that
area with light can feel very secure. Alternatively, creating an
imaginary line of light spiralling upwards and surrounding the
body, then *pinning* it down the centre into the earth is a good
one. One teacher suggested pulling down a roller blind, but the
class at the time felt that cut everything off and would not allow
intuition or healing to work; a variation was suggested of pulling
such a blind upwards from the ground and peeping over the top.
It was a very serious course and we reacted childishly by getting
the giggles, and imagining snuggling into a nice warm sleeping
bag while keeping head in or out according to need. So anything
goes, as long as it makes you feel protected from any harm that
might befall you in this strange territory of the fourth dimension.

Many people feel protected by having an object with them
designated for this purpose. As part of our course we do a
demonstration in the garden: a volunteer has his or her arm
strength tested as a datum, and is then asked to stand on a sink
place — a small area of negative energy which we have located
in advance. Their arm strength is demonstrably weaker, and
everyone is amazed. We are showing why it is not a good idea

to spend time on a place where there is negative earth energy! But one day a student was not affected: he was a strong young man, a fireman, originally from New Zealand, and we congratulated him on being impervious to the effects that were shown to drain everyone else. How did he do it? At first he didn't know, then he took out of his pocket a small wooden object which he called his Tiki, and which represented his tribal totem from his Maori origins. He said it had been given to him for his protection back in his home country, and he never attended a fire without it. It obviously had considerable potency!

Lots of people wear a cross or a crystal or some personal talisman on a chain around their neck, which has been programmed for the same purpose. In the practice of transpersonal psychology, any inner journey is accompanied by such a talisman, whether an actual artefact or visualised in the person's imagination. In this scheme of things not only is it used to provide protection, but it can also be asked for advice and direction at points along the inner journey, so it is helping the person access their own intuition.

Any kind of meditative practice designed to *centre* a person will help them to be stronger in themselves and more focussed on what they are doing. Whether we are working as a couple or facilitating a group for dowsing or healing, we always start with a short time of sitting silently together to allow each person to quieten down from the busyness of their outer lives and enter into the purpose of our meeting. We do this again if an interruption or distraction results in the necessary focus being fragmented. This is not the place for a lesson in meditation, but it doesn't have to be complicated or extended to serve the purpose we need. Among a group attending our initial workshop there are often people who have never tried to meditate, so to help them get *with us* we suggest they just sit comfortably and quietly, and be aware of their surroundings, and that serves very well for starters.

There is another important area of the work when protection is needed: that is, when working on-site. It is advisable to do all the dowsing and most of the standing around answering questions etc., **off** the lines. That is why we needed the map to find out where the lines are before we visit. If you happen to be on a draining earth energy line, you are going to flatten your personal vitality battery much more quickly if you are deliberately engaging with it. In the analogy about the light staying on in the boot of your car, this situation is more like leaving your headlights on while you enjoy dinner with your friends. We know one person who did a huge amount of work in the landscape, and in spite of caring for himself with homoeopathic remedies etc., died of a heart attack. Another friend who was devoted to work in this field, had a heart attack and didn't die, but subsequently had significant psychiatric problems. Neither concerned themselves with concepts of protection.

When Ann experienced her first pinning, on a course with Bruce, she felt the change of energy very strongly in her solar plexus as the stake went in, and was physically sick. Bruce was not sympathetic. 'I thought that might happen,' he said, 'so you have now learned the lesson and need to find a way to protect yourself.' Some lessons are rather messy, it seems! But he had a point. Ann's way is to take the force of the impact on her hand, and immediately rub it into the earth: it works. When doing this healing job on-site, we warn anyone around that they might feel this kind of effect, and make sure they are standing off the lines before driving the stake. But someone has to hold that stake, at least until it is steady in the ground, and someone else has to be on the line wielding the hammer. One day we took our apprentice group of people learning to do this work on a field trip, as a healing was needed very close to our home. The owners were not available so Roy drove the stake. However, one of the students, who volunteered to hold it, felt very peculiar, and needed some personal healing to help him recover. The group discussed the matter (a good lesson of course!) and reckoned that he should have stood at right angles to the flow of the line, not immediately downstream of the stake. So now we gnow.

Certainly there is a need to disconnect, to make a definite

break from being in the dowsing or healing mode after doing this work. Most healers have a ritual for this, and it's usually about washing, especially hands. An acupuncturist told us that the washing should extend up the wrists, to cover important meridians. As usual the ritual itself does not matter, it's the intent behind it which produces the effect. If no water is available, rubbing the hands together vigorously would be helpful. Or visualising a cleansing shower, or an infusion of light all around the body would be another possibility. Roy invented one which involved bringing a mesh (he visualised a tennis racquet!) down from above his head to the ground below his feet, sieving out any negative aspects of what had just been happening around him.

Visualisation

Visualisation is a useful tool in healing, whether of self or others, and can be seen as a positive prayer mechanism. Ann taught it as a self-help tool to patients at the Bristol Cancer Help Centre, as well as to healers. It is a right brain function, which allows access to intuitive and spiritual levels, as well as playing a large part in psychosomatic manifestations, whether damaging or enhancing for the individual. There is often confusion between meditation and visualisation: it is simple to differentiate if you think of meditation as passive, and visualisation as active, mind activity. Meditation is receptive, switches off activity as much as possible, using a simple focus such as the breath or a mantra. Visualisation is active, for instance, a cancer patient would 'see' the tumour leave their body and be disposed of in a way that seemed right to them — the scenario arising from the patient's own psyche is the best in these circumstances. 'See' was written in inverted commas because there is no need for an actual visual image; just so long as the person knows that the image they are working with is there in their mind, no actual pictures are required. Both these states of mind work better if the body is physically relaxed, by which we mean that the muscles are doing as little as possible. Visualisation can be a powerful tool, so care needs to be taken to make sure it is used in a helpful and ethical way. If you are thinking how dreadful someone's illness is when you pray for them or contemplate your own problem, you are likely to do more harm than good: visualising them happy and in good health or yourself with the problem solved would be far more fruitful.

The last consideration we want to mention in this chapter may seem a little strange, but we find it to be valid. Keep the concepts for which you dowse and the methods you use for healing as simple as possible: the more details, artefacts and complications you bring in, the more scope there is for mistakes and distortions. We were told as children, when we asked too many questions 'Curiosity killed the cat'; certainly it can distort accuracy by bringing in irrelevant variables. You only need to find out the minimum of information that enables a healing to be effected. There is no point in finding out more, especially as it is likely to become less accurate. It is our experience that simplicity and single-mindedness make for a better quality of work.

Chapter 10

WHAT NEXT?

Well, we are not fortune-tellers, so we don't know really. But we fully expect Upstairs to send us plenty more learning situations.

One thing seems obvious — judging by the numbers of people asking us for help more are becoming aware of the effects of subtle energies on their lives and health.

The graph below shows the growth of enquiries we have received over the last decade. There is an unusual increase in 1998 due to publicity in *The Sunday Times*, but aside from that the numbers are growing year on year in what looks like an

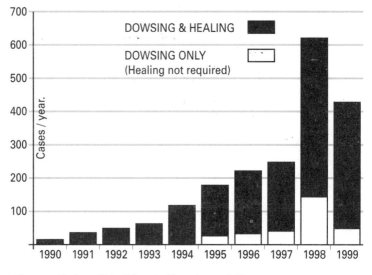

Figure 10.1 — Workload: Number of Cases per year 1990–99

exponential curve. This is in spite of the fact that we do not advertise: most people come to us because a therapist who already knows us or a satisfied client, has put them in touch. We have leaflets and handouts, which hopefully explain things to people who might be interested, or have already contacted us, so that they are clear about what they are asking for before any commitment to partake. We are hoping that our apprentice group, meeting regularly to acquire and improve skills in this work, will produce enough healers of sick houses to meet the need. We are much nearer seventy years of age than sixty, so we won't be able to keep it up for ever!

Meanwhile, we are collaborating with Dr Victoria Wass of Cardiff University in a research project to evaluate the effects of our work. At the time of writing we do not have sufficient data to publish our results but initial findings indicate beneficial effects corresponding to the healing of negative earth energies.

This is the first time that a systematic evaluation of this kind of healing work has been carried out. The purpose is first to establish a statistical effect (i.e. does it work?) and then to explore some of the ways in which it works. We are in the process of surveying 150 households as they approach us (excluding only those who do not need healing), to investigate those who are adversely affected by earth energies and to carry out healing. Each responding household is asked to complete a series of four questionnaires which request information about the characteristics of the household and property, the circumstances of its inhabitants and the nature of the symptoms which are the cause for concern. The first questionnaire is completed in advance of healing, the third and fourth questionnaires are completed afterwards (the latter four weeks afterwards). In this way we are able to compare symptoms before and after our healing work. The timing of the second questionnaire is designed to control for possible placebo effects that we might otherwise attribute to the effects of healing. Half the sample receives the second questionnaire before healing and half afterwards. The experiment is double blind, in that neither the responding household nor the analyst knows which of the second questionnaires have been completed after healing.

In each questionnaire, we include a set of twenty-six questions that capture the spread of symptoms and problems that we have encountered during the course of our healing work. The set of questions is shown in Appendix 3. As well as measuring any improvements that result from healing, these questions allow us to relate symptoms to the characteristics of the house, the circumstances of the household and the results of our dowsing for earth energy effects. As this goes to press the first three questionnaires have been analysed for the first fifty respondents. The results are very promising and are indicative of a definite healing effect.

We asked a doctor who is referring people to us to assess the results on a percentage scale. She measures geopathic stress on a Bicom machine. We have sixteen reports so far, and all but one have been assessed at 90 per cent or more clear after our healing; having registered anything from 30 per cent to 80 per cent before healing.

A kinesiologist offered to carry out a similar before and after test using muscle-testing. She has not been able to provide us with a written report due to pressure of work — it's more important to help people to get better than to write about it! — but announces verbally that all the people she has sent to us (about sixty) test strong on geopathic stress after we have done our work. Can't be bad. We hope to get some figures tabulated before long.

Meanwhile we dowse before and after situations for our own investigations. We prefer to mark scores out of 12, a more significant number, than out of 10 or 100. When 12 is best we are coming up with scores of 9, 10 and 11 after the work. This is for the aggregate situation, which, as you can see in our checklist (Appendix 2) includes a number of items where we are advising the clients to do something themselves, such as place crystals. So at the time we have healed their energy lines and dowsed our score they may not have done all we suggested, thus the scores may get higher later when they have taken our advice. Roy does this particular part of our dowsing, not knowing what the previous score was as Ann is monitoring the notes out of his sight. Presently, when there are more than twenty-four hours in the day, we will go over them and see if they have risen higher after a period of time. Many of them have scored below five before healing — we even had one scoring zero.

We are also trying out the concept of a neighbourhood score, again before and after our work, with the encouragement of our regular healing group. We wonder if our intervention might improve the wider environments of the places we are asked to heal, or whether they will become beacons in dark places. We have not done enough of this to be able to offer any trends, but at least the neighbourhood scores don't usually go down after healing.

We would like to do a more thorough and controlled survey of those very few cases which need more healing weeks or months later. Part of our 'after sales' service is to go through the past year's work at the beginning of each month, dowsing for any that need further attention. We come up with less than one per cent each time, and some of these involve reminding people to cleanse crystals or something simple rather than the re-healing of energy lines which have *gone negative*.

Width and Strength of Lines

From the beginning of our work with Bruce, it was assumed that the width of a line correlated with its strength: that is, that the width could be dowsed on the ground as well as on the map, and the wider it was the greater effect it would have on the people living or working there. We haven't seen any reason to change this assumption to date. We do observe that the lines fluctuate according to the phases of the moon. They dowse wider for full moons and narrower for new moons, very like spring and neap tides. It would be great to make a study of these, dowsing every day, to see if our empirical observations mean anything. A fellow dowser has done a similar study

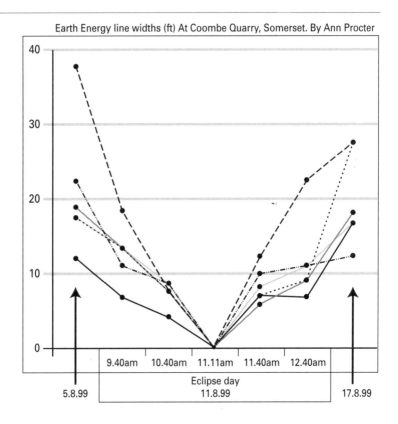

Earth Energy line widths (ft) At Coombe Quarry, Somerset. By Ann Procter

Figure 10.2 — Earth Energy Line Widths on Eclipse Day

relating the strength of earth energy lines surrounding a church: they increase after services (especially at Easter) and after weddings and funerals.

We made some dowsed observations about the width of lines here at our home over the period of the total eclipse of the sun in August 1999. Roy was away on a boat in the English Channel experiencing totality on the day, but co-operated with dowsing the seven lines through our four acres of land 6 days before and 6 days after the event. Ann spent the morning of eclipse day dowsing at home off the lines, and found to her alarm that they went down to zero at totality, but thankfully picked up again later. This was totally unexpected, but correlated with some similar dowsing work undertaken at Avebury. A friend was in Cornwall and found the energy lines where he was dowsing expanded more and more, beyond where he could follow them, but he maintained this was not inconsistent with Ann's findings here at home. Dowsers always do find different results! There is a possible explanation that he was dowsing the way the lines were relating to the moon which was taking the upper hand, and Ann was relating them to the sun which was covered over. Who knows?

There are many wonders to be explored. We do hope we have time to look into more of them before our dotage sets in. Do enjoy making your own investigations.

Appendix 1

Resources

The National Federation of Spiritual Healers
Old Manor Farm Studio
Church Street, Sunbury-on-Thames
Middlesex TW16 6RG
Tel: 01932 783164
Fax: 01932 779648
Healer Referral Service Tel: 0891 616080
Web site: www.nfsh.org.uk
E-mail: office@nfsh.org.uk

The British Society of Dowsers
Sycamore Barn, Hastingleigh
Ashford, Kent TN25 5HW
Tel/Fax: 01233 750253
Web site: www.dowsers.demon.co.uk

Earth Energy Group of the British Society of Dowsers
Mrs Jo Cartmale
Secretary/Treasurer
16 Woodland Walk, Billing Lane
Northampton NN3 5NS

The Feng Shui Society
377 Edgware Road
London W2 1BT
Tel: 07050 289 200
Web site: www.fengshuisociety.org.uk

The American Society of Dowsers
101 Railroad Street, St Johnsbury
Vermont 05819 USA
Tel: (802) 748-8565 and (800) 711-9497
Fax: (802) 684-2565

The Bristol Cancer Help Centre
Grove House, Cornwallis Grove
Clifton, Bristol BS8 4PG
Tel: 0117 980 9500
Fax: 0117 923 9184
E-mail: info@bristolcancerhelp.org.uk

The College of Psychic Studies
16 Queensberry Place
London SW7 2EB
Tel: 020 7589 3293
Fax: 020 7589 2824

Geomancy MagEzine
Good articles, information and references.
Web site: www.geomancy.org

Dowsing Courses and Healing Sick Houses
Roy and Ann Procter
Coombe Quarry
Keinton Mandeville
near Somerton
Somerset TA11 6DQ
Tel: 0148 223215
Fax: 0148 224234
E-mail: procter@dial.pipex.com
Web site: www.dspace.dial.pipex.com/procter

Scientific and Medical Network
Lake House
Vann Lake Road
Ockley
Lower Dorking, Surrey RH5 5NS
Tel: 01306 710072
Fax: 01306 710073
Web site: www.cis.plym.ac.uk/SciMedNet.home.htm
E-mail: scimednetwork@compuserve.com

Appendix 2

Our Dowsing Checklist

	dates	
First Enquiry:		
Dowse Address:		Name:
Map Diagnosis:		Address:
Treatment:		
Check req. by us:		
		phone:
Check req. by client:		ref:
Donation:		
LINES: number:		
+ve:		
−ve:		
additional sinks:		
additional fountains:		
ENTITIES:		place related:
		person related:
		helpful:
		unhelpful:
POWER OBJECTS		helpful:
		unhelpful:
ADVERSE EFFECTS from		
domestic electricity:		
internal microwaves:		
external microwaves:		
domestic water:		internal:
		external:
loose water:		chemical:
		informational:
airborne gases:		
SCORES OUT OF 12		
aggregates:		
neighbourhood:		
OTHER:		
Notes:		

Appendix 3

Questionnaire Used In Our Research Project

For each of the conditions listed below, please circle the number that describes most accurately the experience of the chosen person over the **last week.**

If you have not experienced the condition, please circle '0' and do not complete the rest of the line.

		Not exper- ienced	To a mild degree	To a mod- erate degree	To an intense degree	A little of the time	Some of the time	A good deal of the time	Most of the time	All the time
A	Lack of interest and motivation	0	1	2	3	1	2	3	4	5
B	Suffer from repeated infections	0	1	2	3	1	2	3	4	5
C	Downhearted and low	0	1	2	3	1	2	3	4	5
D	Calm and peaceful	0	1	2	3	1	2	3	4	5
E	Full of life and vitality	0	1	2	3	1	2	3	4	5
F	Physically worn down	0	1	2	3	1	2	3	4	5
G	Mentally worn down	0	1	2	3	1	2	3	4	5
H	Lack of energy	0	1	2	3	1	2	3	4	5
I	Problems with neighbours	0	1	2	3	1	2	3	4	5
J	Worried about health	0	1	2	3	1	2	3	4	5
K	Worried about home	0	1	2	3	1	2	3	4	5
L	Happy and contented	0	1	2	3	1	2	3	4	5
M	Trouble sleeping	0	1	2	3	1	2	3	4	5
N	Bad dreams	0	1	2	3	1	2	3	4	5
O	Strange happenings at home	0	1	2	3	1	2	3	4	5
P	Problems at work	0	1	2	3	1	2	3	4	5
Q	Optimistic	0	1	2	3	1	2	3	4	5
R	Worried about money	0	1	2	3	1	2	3	4	5
S	Unsettled at home	0	1	2	3	1	2	3	4	5
T	Anxious and tense	0	1	2	3	1	2	3	4	5
U	Generally troubled	0	1	2	3	1	2	3	4	5
V	Problems with electrical equipment	0	1	2	3	1	2	3	4	5
W	Domestic harmony	0	1	2	3	1	2	3	4	5
X	Bad atmosphere at home	0	1	2	3	1	2	3	4	5
Y	Difficult relationships	0	1	2	3	1	2	3	4	5
Z	Bad luck	0	1	2	3	1	2	3	4	5

Please add anything that you think would be of interest.

Glossary

Aura: The subtle body enveloping the physical body.

Black Stream: An earth energy line with harmful qualities. Also, a term used by water dowsers to denote an underground stream that is not considered potable.

Chakra: Vital force centre. An interconnection point between the subtle and physical bodies.

Energy: Throughout this book the word *energy* has been used as in earth energy and healing energy etc. (*See* Authors' Note, p. xiv)

Earth Energy: A naturally occurring field of subtle energy relating to, or emanating from, the earth as a whole.

Fountain: An earth energy spot with beneficial qualities.

Fourth Dimension: Colloquial term for subtle levels beyond our physical awareness.

Geopathic Stress: Medically accepted term for depleting earth energies.

ME: Myalgic Encephalomyelitis. A disease whose diagnosis is controversial among the medical profession; generally results in lack of energy, aching limbs and susceptibility to infections. We refer to it as *muddled energies* or *flat battery disease.*

Paradigm: Pattern or concept.

Parameter: A quantity or measurement.

Power Object: Some object that has an *energy* or powerful association attached to it.

Sacred Site: A location where the veil between the physical and *other* states of being are less opaque. A place of powerful earth energies, usually beneficial unless they have become contaminated.

Sink Place: An earth energy spot with harmful qualities.

Subtle: When used in this book, denotes the non-physical worlds.

Transpersonal Psychology: Psychology with a soul: recognises the existence of intuitive and spiritual levels of awareness.

Trendle: Part of a sacred site usually used for special dances to enhance beneficial energies, e.g. maypole dancing. Sited at a significant point in the earth energy pattern.

Bibliography and References

This reading list has been prepared to assist in your further studies. Just giving a list of titles and authors is not always very helpful — how do you choose? So we have written short notes on each book from our own reading. We have done this to help you decide the ones that you might wish to read for yourself.

It is divided into sections of interest but some of the books do not fit neatly into the sections! Thus, there is some overlap and the sections chosen can only be a rough guide.

Some books are especially recommended and are starred:
* Recommended
** Highly Recommended — *Must Read!*

Section 1: Dowsing

1.1 Graves, T., *The Dowsers Workbook*, Turnstone Press: 1976. Aquarian: 1989.
   * A good comprehensive and practical book. Undogmatic!
1.2 Lonegren, S., *The Pendulum Kit*, Simon & Schuster: 1990.
   * A relatively expensive book but the pack does contain a very nice responsive brass pendulum. Useful book with some interesting applications detailed.
1.3 Lonegren, S., *The Dowsing Rod Kit*, Eddison Sadd: 1995.
   * Another Kit. This one contains a pair of dowsing angle rods, some pegs as markers, a notepad and an excellent book with contributions by various people.
1.4 Lonegren, S., *Spiritual Dowsing*, Gothic Image: 1996.
   ** Our favourite book on dowsing. This is the nearest to the way we see it and the way we teach dowsing on our courses.
1.5 Ozaniec, N., *Dowsing for Beginners*, Hodder & Stoughton: 1994. Very good, undogmatic.
1.6 Ross, T.E. and Wright, R.D., *The Divining Mind*, Destiny: 1990.
   * By instructors from the American Society of Dowsers. We do not agree with the rigid progression of skills taught in this book, but there's some very useful material here and the methods taught will suit some people.
(*See also* 7.1 and 7.2 which have useful chapters on dowsing.)

Section 2: Other States of Existence

This section gives clues to states of existence other than the *on earth, physical* with which we are all familiar. Different people have different perceptions, depending very often on their own belief systems. Thus, it is useful to compare a number of different books and decide for yourself what you think!

2.1   Cannon, D., *Conversations With Nostradamus*, vols 1, 2 and 3, Ozark Mountain: 1992.
      Direct two-way conversations with Nostradamus across time. He explains what he was trying to convey and why he had to conceal it the way he did. Really makes you think about the nature of time apart from authoritative exposition of the quatrains by the original author.

2.2   Cannon, D., *Jesus and the Essenes*, Gateway Books: 1992.
      Same process as the book above. Discussions with a member of the Essene community at the time of Jesus, who studied within the community. Valuable eye witness accounts of Jesus and events of the time. Includes beliefs of the community members and indicates Jesus's message which has been somewhat modified by religious leaders since.

2.3   Cannon, D., *Between Death and Life*, Gateway Books: 1993.
      * Fascinating insights into our state of existence between incarnations on earth, obtained by hypnotic regression. A number of different views are presented from which a common thread can be perceived. Dolores Cannon would seem to be a very gifted practitioner in this field.

2.4   Johnson, R.C., *The Imprisoned Splendour*, Hodder & Stoughton: 1965.
      A seminal book for us. A scientist's view of other states of awareness.

2.5   IO'Sullivan, T. and O'Sullivan, N., *Soul Rescuers: A 21st Century Guide to the Spirit World*, Thorsons: 1999.
      This recent publication contains much good information on those in the spirit world and their interaction with our own physical existence. Some of this interaction can be very unhelpful to us. The O'Sullivans have looked at people's attitude to physical death and preparations for the next state of existence within a variety of different cultures, often much different to our own. Also described are a number of cases in which the O'Sullivans have been able to solve the resulting problems. They indicate their method of working, which may be fine for them, but we would caution others from using their methods, or attempting

any of this work without very competent instruction and supervision by a reliable and experienced teacher.

2.6   Richelieu, P., *A Soul's Journey*, Turnstone Press: 1972. Aquarian: 1989.

* This is an account of a strange series of visits from an Indian gentleman, of mysterious origin, who takes the author on a series of *journeys* to a graduated series of planes of existence.

2.7   Sandys, Lady C. and Lehmann, R., *The Awakening Letters*, vol. 1, Neville Spearman: 1978.

2.8   Sandys, Lady C. and Lehmann, R., *The Awakening Letters*, vol. 2, C.W. Daniel: 1986.

* The above two books are all channelled by Cynthia, Lady Sandys from her relatives or very close friends. We knew Cynthia and Father Andrew Glazewski (one of those who communicates) and can vouch for the integrity of those involved. Father Andrew describes in detail his own death from a heart attack. It has been interesting to compare his account with that of those present at the time.

2.9   Tudor Pole, W., *Writing on the Ground*, Neville Spearman: 1968.

2.10   Tudor Pole, W., *The Silent Road*, Neville Spearman: 1978.

2.11   Tudor Pole, W., *My Dear Alexias: Letters from Wellesley Tudor Pole to Rosamond Lehmann*, Neville Spearman: 1979.

2.12   Tudor Pole, W. and Lehmann, R., *A Man Seen Afar*, Neville Spearman: 1983.

* The above four books are all the thoughts of the remarkable modern seer Wellesley Tudor Pole. They deal with many significant events throughout his life. He presents his experiences in a humble and non-dogmatic way. He insists that you only accept those things that seem right to you. The references 2.9 and 2.12 give a number of his *on-the-spot* visions of parts of the life of Jesus. These were obtained by what he calls *far memory*, and are very interesting. The collection of letters in reference 2.11, *My Dear Alexias*, give many insights into his perceptions, including much of the development of the Chalice Well Trust.

2.13   Whitton, Dr J., *Life Between Life*, Grafton: 1987.

* A very interesting account of a number of cases in which subjects have been regressed to previous lives. The special aspect of this book is that the subjects also describe the periods between their physical lives and show the relevance of these memories to their earthly lives.

Section 3: Relevant *Science*

This section contains books which try to explain things on some sort of organised scientific basis. However, many scientists would not consider all the books listed here sufficiently rigorous. Nevertheless, they do provide valuable food for thought and one day their ideas may become sufficiently developed to be accepted as conventional wisdom!

3.1   Alexandersson, O., *Living Water: Viktor Schauberger and the Secrets of Natural Energy*, Gateway Books: 1990.
A small and readable book on the life and work of Victor Schauberger. He developed remarkable theories on the properties of water by long observation of mountain streams. This led to his discovery of implosion energy, a natural free energy process yet to be properly exploited.

3.2   Ash, D. and Hewitt, P., *Science of the Gods*, Gateway Books: 1990. (Now retitled as *The Vortex.*)
* A look at the basis of matter. A new view of Lord Kelvin's vortex theory of the nature of matter. The authors develop this concept by suggesting that there can be many different types of matter depending on the speed of the creating wave motion. Thus, everything in our material universe is formed by waves that travel at speeds not exceeding that of light. Some waves seem to travel faster than the speed of light and form a different sort of matter with different properties.

3.3   Bergsmann, O., *Risk Factor: Place, Dowsing Zone and Man*, University Publishing House Facultas: Vienna 1990.
(Scientific study investigating place-related influences in man. In German, £28.)
We have only had an incomplete synopsis explained to us by a German-speaking friend as there is not yet an English translation. It is a most comprehensive and respectable research project, funded by the Austrian Government, involving medical institutions. 'It shows without a doubt the negative influence of geopathic stress zones, or black streams, on human health.' (Quote from *Journal of the British Society of Dowsers*, March 1993.) The investigations continue and we 'stay tuned'.

3.4   Coats, C., *Living Energies*, Gateway Books: 1996.
A full and detailed presentation of Schauberger's work, probably the most complete yet made. We have to say we found this book *hard going*. An invaluable work for the seriously interested.

3.5   Cowan, D. and Girdlestone, R., *Safe as Houses? Ill-Health and Electro-Stress in the Home*, Gateway Books: 1996.

** There are not many books on geopathic stress, earth energies etc. with which we wholeheartedly concur. However, this is by far the best and most comprehensive one on the subject we have yet seen and we have little with which to quibble.

3.6 Hall, A., *Water, Electricity and Health*, Hawthorn Press: 1997.
This excellent book gives the results of Alan's research into the life form information stored within the microstructure of water. This information is vital for all living things and is being corrupted, mainly by man-made electrical and microwaves sources. Alan describes the effect of this information corruption and the methods he has developed to help correct the situation, a matter of importance to us all.

3.7 Hertel, H. et al, *Hidden Hazards of Microwave Cooking*, Nexus, No. 25, April–May: 1995.
Magazine article reporting on the research by Hans Hertel et al and the consequent attempt to suppress their findings.

3.8 Merz, B., *Points of Cosmic Energy*, C.W. Daniel: 1987.
Here is a very comprehensive survey of earth energy lines at a wide variety of places in various parts of the world and their effects. The work is spoilt by the great detail and the numerical field strengths quoted, based on dowsing against a scale of numbers (Bovis Biometer). These figures are highly individual to the dowser and of no absolute significance.

3.9 Oldfield, H. and Coghill, R., *The Dark Side of the Brain*, Element Books: 1988.
An important book suggesting that the human body control systems are electrically based rather than chemically based. This is supported by results of Kirlian photography and the considerable success that Oldfield has obtained with electrocrystal therapy. Oldfield has recently developed equipment that enables the *energy body* to be viewed in motion by video. This must be one of the most significant diagnostic tools ever invented.

3.10 Pohl, G.F. von, *Earth Currents: Causative Factor of Cancer and Other Diseases*, Frech-Verlag: 1987.
This is a modern translation of the book originally published in Germany in 1932. It sets out the detailed work carried out by von Pohl into the effect of earth energies on health. He does not deal with the change of quality of energy, his solution is always to move the furniture or move house. If you can put up with his assertion that adverse earth energies are responsible for everything, this is a valuable piece of work.

3.11 Schiff, M., *The Memory of Water: Homoeopathy and the Battle of Ideas in the New Sciences*, Thorsons: 1998. (Concerns the work of Benveniste.)

Section 4: The Meaning of Life

These books, we believe, are of very great significance. They have been very important to us in the development of what, we hope, is understanding of the significance of our existence and our relationship to the universe.

4.1   Cousins, D., *A Handbook for Light Workers*, Barton House: 1993.
      * This is a very useful book, giving guidance on coping with the new energies manifesting on the planet at this time, and how to assist the developments in mankind. There is much explanatory material on the nature of our existence and our relationship with other states of being. The book includes many meditations for a wide variety of situations where *energy changes* may be required. While wholeheartedly commending this book, we think some of the detail is not necessarily as absolute as it is presented. Therefore, do not take it all at face value, but use it to build up your own process as seems right to you.

4.2   Mason, P. and Laing, R., *Sai Baba, The Embodiment of Love*, Gateway Books: 1993.
      ** This book had a profound effect on Roy. He now thinks that Sai Baba is the divinity incarnate, and is probably the *Second Coming* incarnation that Christians expect. Two people of considerable experience write this book with great sincerity. There are other books about Sai Baba that would seem to support this view.

4.3   Mazzoleni, M., *A Catholic Priest Meets Sai Baba*, Leela Press: 1993.
      This is the story of an investigation of Sai Baba by a Roman Catholic priest as part of his own spiritual quest. He concludes, as many others have done, that Sai Baba is a most remarkable person and is what he claims to be. Unfortunately his findings were not well received by the Church and he was excommunicated.

4.4   Redfield, J., *The Celestine Prophecy*, Warner Books: 1993.

4.5   Redfield, J., *The Tenth Insight*, Bantam Books: 1996.
      The above two publications are excellent books in story form helping to crystallise perceptions of *why you are where you are* in life. *The Tenth Insight* follows on from *The Celestine Prophecy* but could be read first on its own.

4.6   Schlemmer, P. and Jenkins, P., *The Only Planet of Choice: Essential Briefings from Deep Space*, Gateway Books: 1993. (There is a later, revised version)
      ** This is a distillation of twenty years of channelled wisdom from a very high source known as *The Nine*. Don't miss it!

Section 5: Sacred Geometry

5.1 Graves, T., *Needles of Stone Revisited*, Gothic Image: 1986.
* This is a reissue of the original *Needles of Stone*, published in 1978 by Turnstone. It is a very thought-provoking book and one of the earliest to deal with earth energies, their relationship with old stone circles, standing stones etc., and their effect on every-day life now.
5.2 Michell, J., *The New View Over Atlantis*, Thames & Hudson: 1983.
* This excellent book is a good introduction to some of the principles of sacred geometry and its application as visible in landscape and buildings. A good place to start on this subject.
5.3 Miller, H. and Broadhurst, P., *The Sun and The Serpent*, Pendragon: 1990.
Describes the authors' dowsing journey tracking the *Michael and Mary* earth energy lines from south-west England through to the Norfolk coast.

Section 6: Healing

A large number of books have been written on this subject; we have only noted ones of special value from our own point of view.

6.1 Bailey, A., *Dowsing For Health*, Quantum (Foulsham): 1990.
* Covers the application of dowsing to health and healing by one of the acknowledged experts in this field.
6.2 Benor, Dr D.J., *Holistic Energy Medicine and Spirituality*, vol. 1, Helix: 1993.
A thorough investigation into healing research.
6.3 Brennan, B.A., *Hands of Light: A Guide to Healing Through the Human Energy Field*, Bantam: 1988.
* Inspiring book dealing with energy fields in the Human Aura, with masses of pictures. Surprisingly inexpensive.
6.4 Featherstone, Dr C. and Forsyth, L., *Medical Marriage*, Findhorn Press: 1997.
This book is helping to develop a partnership between orthodox and complementary medicine. It is very comprehensive, in that it contains details of over sixty complementary therapies and their applicability. These are written by experts in their particular fields. (We contributed the section on dowsing.) There are plenty of references and lists for further reading. A comprehensive and valuable book for healthcare professionals and others.
6.5 MacManaway, B., *Healing, The Energy that can Restore Health*, Thorsons: 1983.
** A valuable and significant book for us because it was written by one of the country's most notable healers.

6.6 Meares, A., *The Wealth Within*, Ashgrove: 1986.
     A masterpiece introducing meditation.
6.7 Simonton, O.C., Mathews-Simonton, S. and Creighton, J., *Getting Well Again*, J. Tarcher Inc: 1978.
     Pioneered the use of visualisation in *self-help in cancer.*
6.8 St Aubyn, L., ed., *Healing*, Heinemann: 1983.
     Several essays by people who *know their stuff*. Valuable for its good bibliography.

Section 7: Psychic Protection

This is a very important subject for anyone getting into dowsing, healing etc. We need to be aware of the dangers involved in opening up to other states of consciousness.

7.1 Bloom, W., *Psychic Protection*, Piatkus: 1997.
     ** A very readable book by an author well respected in this field.
7.2 Hall, J., *The Art of Psychic Protection*, Findhorn Press: 1996.
     ** We have known Judy personally for many years and have had experience of her work, which is first class in every respect.

Section 8: Psychology

8.1 Assagioli, R., *Psychosynthesis*, Turnstone Books: 1965.
     Core work on transpersonal psychology and the egg diagram.
8.2 Cade, C.M. and Coxhead, N., *The Awakened Mind*, Delacorte Press/Eleanor Friede; 1979.
     Biofeedback and the development of higher states of awareness.

Section 9: Subtle Anatomy

9.1 Rendel, P., *Introduction to the Chakras*, Aquarian: 1986.
     A very simple introduction.
9.2 Roney-Dougal, Dr S., *Where Science and Magic Meet*, Element: 1991.
     Excellent review of the chakras in Chapter 4.
9.3 Tansley, D., *Subtle Body*, Thames & Hudson: 1977.
     Thorough and pictorial review of the chakra system.

Section 10: Additional Material

10.1 Lonegren, S. and MacManaway, Dr P., eds., *Mid Atlantic Geomancy*.
     This is a magazine published on the internet with interesting articles on dowsing, *earth mysteries*, labyrinths etc. Web site is at www.geomancy.org

About the Authors

Roy, born 1930, is a retired Chartered Engineer, a Fellow of the Royal Aeronautical Society, with a long career in the design of transport aircraft, and practical piloting skills. He has constructional hobbies, making anything from models of all kinds, including steam locomotives to life-size gliders, aeroplanes and boats. He is also skilled in practical building and repair jobs. He now enjoys sailing.

Ann, born 1932, is a doctor's daughter with a wide range of skills and qualifications, used in self-employed work. Her university career was ended in serious illness, deemed terminal when diagnosed, so she has a degree in 'life and death' rather than the usual paper qualification. Past involvement in antenatal and stress management teaching groups led on to further training and to a job as a social worker in a psychiatric hospital. She then trained in counselling, psychotherapy and psychological astrology, and is now accredited by the British Association for Counselling and registered with the United Kingdom Council of Psychotherapists. She manages a large garden and keeps bees.

Both Roy and Ann are registered healers with the National Federation of Spiritual Healers and on the register of the British Society of Dowsers. They are both Trustees of the Chalice Well in Glastonbury, Roy being Chairman.

Their two daughters have produced five grandchildren, and Ann also acts under an Enduring Power of Attorney for her very elderly mother.

Index